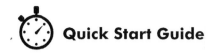 **Quick Start Guide**

D1434859

The Essential
THYROID DIET
RECIPE BOOK

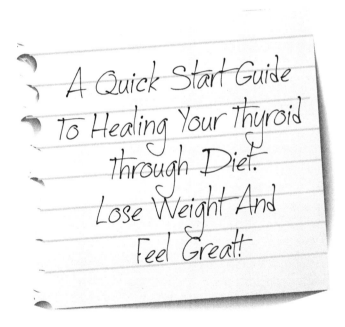

A Quick Start Guide To Healing Your Thyroid through Diet. Lose Weight And Feel Great!

With Delicious Thyroid Friendly Recipes

First published in 2017 by Erin Rose Publishing

Text and illustration copyright © 2017 Erin Rose Publishing

Design: Julie Anson

ISBN: 978-1-911492-14-6

A CIP record for this book is available from the British Library.

DISCLAIMER: This book is for informational purposes only and not intended as a substitute for the medical advice, diagnosis or treatment of a physician or qualified healthcare provider. The reader should consult a physician before undertaking a new health care regime and in all matters relating to his/her health, and particularly with respect to any symptoms that may require diagnosis or medical attention.

While every care has been taken in compiling the recipes for this book we cannot accept responsibility for any problems which arise as a result of preparing one of the recipes. The author and publisher disclaim responsibility for any adverse effects that may arise from the use or application of the recipes in this book. Some of the recipes in this book include nuts and eggs. If you have an egg or nut allergy it's important to avoid these. It is recommended that children, pregnant women, the elderly or anyone who has an immune system disorder avoid eating raw eggs.

CONTENTS

Recipes

Lunch

Dinner

Snacks & Sweet Treats 93

INTRODUCTION

Can't lose weight? Tired and feeling the cold? You could have an underactive thyroid and not be aware of it! An underactive thyroid, also known as hypothyroidism, is one of the most commonly undiagnosed and misdiagnosed diseases in the UK. Millions of people worldwide are affected yet they have no explanation for their symptoms such as fatigue and weight gain.

Statistics show an increasing incidence of thyroid disease and there is conflicting opinion as to whether this is down to improved diagnosis or whether thyroid disease is almost becoming epidemic.

So many people are looking for ways to improve the effectiveness of their thyroid and achieve optimal health. There are various causes of hypothyroidism, which we will look at, together with how changing your diet and improving your nutrition can really improve your health and vitality.

In this **Quick Start Guide**, we provide you with the essential information you need to take control and boost your thyroid health and improve your lifestyle. By making some changes to your daily routine, you can improve your weight, vitality and maximise your health.

In this comprehensive book we not only tell you what foods can harm and heal your thyroid but we bring you plenty of simple and delicious every day recipes which make healthy eating a real treat. If you suspect your thyroid is an issue or if you have been diagnosed with hypothyroidism and you are ready to improve your well-being, read on!

What Is Thyroid Disease?

Firstly, let's look at what the thyroid is and what it can do for you! The thyroid is a small butterfly-shaped gland located in the Adam's apple area of the neck. It may be small but it is often referred to as the 'master gland' of the body and is a power house which regulates essential functions. The thyroid gland produces T3 and T4 hormones which control metabolism, temperature, heart rate and brain function. When the thyroid gland is working optimally, all is well and bodily functions are normal but when it over or under produces hormones, that's when problems occur.

As you know, the under functioning of the thyroid gland is called hypothyroidism and the symptoms of insufficient thyroid hormone production are:

- Weight gain despite eating normally
- Frequently feeling cold
- Depression, brain fog and muddled thinking
- Fatigue
- Hair loss and coarse, dry hair
- Dry skin
- Stiffness and muscle cramps
- Inflammation
- Constipation
- Low libido
- Palpitations
- Dizziness
- Hair loss of the outer edge of the eyebrow
- Dry eyes
- Fluid retention
- Infertility

Hyprothyroidism is much more common in women than men and it's not uncommon for a hyper functioning thyroid to become under active. In this book we mainly deal with how to improve your underactive thyroid but note that some causes contribute to either condition.

What Causes Hypothyroidism?

- Genetics can mean you have a predisposition to thyroid disease.
- Toxins, heavy metals, pesticides and chemicals which are in the food supply and in the environment have been strongly linked to thyroid disease.
- Mercury from dental fillings entering the body can adversely affect the thyroid.
- Iodine deficiency can lead to an underactive thyroid. If you choose to supplement your iodine intake the maximum recommended intake is no more than 1000mcg a day as excessive amounts can lead to overactive thyroid.
- Mineral deficiencies such as zinc and magnesium.
- Having treatment for hyperthyroid, such as surgery or radioactive iodine can lead to an underactive thyroid.
- Hashimoto's disease, an autoimmune disease, where antibodies are released against the thyroid gland, is considered to be a major cause of hypothyroidism.
- Hypothyroidism affects mostly women and often comes to light during hormonal changes such as the menopause.
- Smoking also increases the risk of developing a thyroid disorder.
- Excessive stress takes its toll on the body and in particular it affects the adrenal glands and their production of the hormone cortisol which can play havoc with the endocrine system and the levels of all hormones in your body, resulting in thyroid problems.

The symptoms of hyperthyroidism or an over functioning thyroid are:
- Unexplained weight loss despite eating normally.
- Insomnia.
- Anxiety.
- Raised heart rate.

What Causes Hyperthyroid?
- Graves' disease, which is a genetic disorder.
- Overmedication causing an underactive thyroid to over stimulate.
- Nodules or lumps on the thyroid causing excessive production of hormones.

Although this book mainly deals with how to deal with an underactive thyroid, it's worth knowing about the other side of the coin as it may be relevant to you and detoxification of mercury is still beneficial.

How To Improve Your Thyroid Health

You may have been under the impression that nothing can be done to naturally improve your symptoms but take heart and know that you can take control of your well-being. The aim of this book is to guide you to improve your health naturally and here is what you can do:

Reduce inflammation in the body.

Improve your diet and correct nutritional deficiencies.

Balance your hormones naturally and healthily.

Reduce your stress levels.

Improve your immune system to better deal with viral and bacterial load.

These are all factors which influence your thyroid function and by taking positive steps, changing your diet and lifestyle and improving these fundamental issues you can feel better!

> **Before you embark on any new dietary or fitness regime always check with your doctor or health professional that it is safe for you to do so, especially if you are on medication which may need to be monitored and/or adjusted. Likewise, if you have symptoms of weight loss, changes to heart rate and any persistent symptoms you should seek medical attention straight away.**

Mercury Overload And How To Detox

Mercury is a heavy metal and toxic substance which can be found in our food chain and is a global cause for concern. Once mercury is in the environment it can easily spread between water, land and air. It is ingested from plankton by fish and birds, increasing in concentration and accumulating in high levels in older and larger fish. Communities which exist mainly on seafood are at a greater risk of mercury toxicity and its harmful effects on the nervous system, brain, lungs, liver and kidneys. Furthermore, it's known that exposure to mercury can have a detrimental effect on the brain development of unborn children and the FDA advise pregnant and breastfeeding women to avoid fish with a high mercury content to protect brain and heart health.

In ancient times mercury was mined by prisoners and slaves and in recent history, mercury was used in the production of felt which was used to make hats. This exposure and toxicity resulted in severe mental disorders and dementia and the term 'mad as a hatter' was born. It was traditionally used in cosmetics, paints, vaccinations, blood pressure monitors and thermometers. Thankfully, products made in the EU have been banned from containing mercury but its use has not been phased out and this is still used in dental fillings, which is a controversial topic.

Mercury has been used in dental fillings for decades and the safety of this practice is still hotly debated with many people opting for alternative types of fillings. Mercury vapours from amalgam fillings can leak into our bodies and continually pose a great threat to our health. The process of extracting the dental filling can increase any leakage from the mercury into the body so it needs to be carried out by a suitably qualified dentist who will take precautions. As to whether you should have your old amalgam fillings extracted, is a personal choice and one directed by the severity of your symptoms and health. If you choose to have the old mercury fillings removed, never have more than one changed at one time to allow your body to process it and make sure your dentist takes specific precautions to prevent any of the old fillings fragmenting, coming loose and being ingested further.

The good news is that you can reduce and eliminate mercury from your body and avoid further exposure. You can still eat fish and it is a great source of iodine and omega oil so getting a supply of nutrients by eating smaller and younger fish with low levels of mercury. If however you are pregnant or breastfeeding it might be best avoided.

Purchasing beauty products online or abroad? You may want to check that your cosmetics do not contain mercury so check the ingredients list for; mercuric, mercurio, mercurous chloride and calomel. It is more often found in anti-aging creams and skin lightening products, particularly in African or Asian countries but even in the UK some creams find their way onto the market, so make sure you aren't unwittingly absorbing mercury from your products. In the US it's recommended such products are avoided and a ban may soon come into place.

Mercury Detox

Eating an abundance of fresh fruits containing pectin is a great way to remove mercury from the body. Pectin is a type of fibre which clears toxins and waste products from the body and has been proven to quickly improve elimination of mercury within 24 hours.

It's really important to eliminate as much mercury as possible as it binds to the thyroid, in a similar way to iodine, but the mercury blocks the iodine which is essential for optimum thyroid functioning.

Adding coriander (cilantro) to your diet will help with the elimination of heavy metals and in particular, mercury. Eat it daily. You can add it to smoothies and adding a handful of fresh coriander leaves to smoothies containing pectin rich fruits such as apples, pears and oranges will increase the detoxification process.

Developing a goitre, an enlarged thyroid gland, indicated by a swelling on the neck is a sign that you have insufficient iodine. If you are in the US you will find much of the salt has iodine added but that isn't the case in the UK. You can increase your iodine levels with a supplement but don't overdo it as to much could over stimulate your thyroid gland. Seaweeds are a great natural and easily digested way to boost your iodine levels and they contain lots of minerals and vitamins too!

Foods To Avoid

Cook fresh whole foods where possible and avoid processed foods. They can contain hidden sugars, harmful fats, sodium, artificial sweeteners and additives like MSG.

- Avoid all fish with high mercury content. These are generally larger and therefore older fish which have ingested mercury over time, especially tuna, shark, swordfish, sea bass and grouper.

- Steer clear of sugar as it disrupts the hormones and metabolism so it's best to avoid all products containing sugar, such as; biscuits, cakes chocolate bars, sweets and candy sweet fizzy drinks, cordials and concentrated juices, sauces, marinades, relishes and dips containing sugar, breakfast cereals, muesli and granola bars containing sugar and/or syrup.

- Avoid gluten which can cause the release of antibodies against the thyroid, particularly if you have known Hashimoto's disease, therefore steer clear of products containing: wheat, barley, rye, semolina, couscous and oats such as pasta, cakes, crackers, biscuits, gravies and sauces containing gluten as a thickener.

- Dairy produce not only contains hormones but they can be inflammatory to the body, even in those who are not lactose intolerant, so products like milk, cheese and cream are best avoided.

- Coffee and tea contain caffeine which is a stimulant and can affect the adrenal glands and blood sugar so it's best avoided.

- Be wary of soya, soya milk and soya products such as tofu, can also interfere with thyroid production and cause iodine deficiency.

Foods You Can Eat

Fish:

Salmon	Hake
Mackerel	Sole
Haddock	Pollock
Talipa	Crayfish
Prawns (shrimps)	Trout
Scallops	Squid
Crab	Sardines
Herring	

All meats and poultry:

Chicken	Turkey
Beef	Pork
Lamb	

Carbohydrates:

Potatoes	Millet
Rice (preferably brown)	Oats (if gluten free)
Sweet potatoes	
Quinoa	

Dairy alternatives:

Almond Milk	Rice Milk
Coconut Milk	Hemp Milk
Coconut Cream	

Vegetables:

Avocados	Sweet potatoes
Broccoli	Spring onions (scallions)
Cauliflower	Spinach
Celery	Leeks
Celeriac	Cabbage
Tomatoes	Pak choy (bok choi)
Courgette (zucchini)	Garlic
Swede	Fresh and dried herbs, like basil,
Lettuce	rosemary, coriander (cilantro),
Cucumber	chives, parsley, lemon balm and
Onions	mint.
Squash	

All spices including:

Turmeric	Ginger
Cumin	Mustard
Paprika	Curry
Pepper	Cinnamon
Chilli	Nutmeg

All fruits including:

Apples	Grapes
Bananas	Lemons
Blackberries	Limes
Blueberries	Pears
Cranberries	Raspberries
Oranges	Redcurrants
Kiwi	Strawberries

Papaya	Dried fruit such as figs, dates,
Mango	prunes, raisins, sultans, mangoes
Pineapple	and bananas in moderation due
	to its higher sugar content. It may
	also have sugar added.

Nuts and seeds including:

Brazil nuts	Pecan nuts
Almonds	Cashews
Chia seeds	Sunflower seeds
Hazelnuts	Pumpkin seeds
Peanuts	Sesame seeds
Walnuts	Flaxseeds/linseeds

Top Foods For Your Thyroid

Blueberries

These delicious berries are loaded with antioxidants and the University of Maryland Medical Centre found they are helpful for hypothyroidism. Blueberries contain the highest amount of inflammation busting and immune boosting antioxidants, so add these to your shopping basket!

Cherries

Once again cherries come out top when it comes to vital nutrients and antioxidants. They've been used to successfully treat gout and their natural anti-inflammatory properties and vitamins aid the thyroid and immune system, helping to protect the body from diseases.

Spirulina

Spirulina, which is a blue-green algae, available in tablet of powder form, has earned itself the reputation of being a true superfood! It contains an abundance of essential amino acids, beta-carotene, B12, calcium iron and many other valuable nutrients. It's a powerful antioxidant, cleanser, detoxifier and gives your energy a large boost. Spirulina is also a natural appetite suppressant and helps reduce inflammation as it balances Ph levels in the body. Hawaiian spirulina is free from pesticides and is the purest form.

Maca

Maca contains B vitamins, iron and zinc which aids the pituitary gland in regulating thyroid hormones.

Squash

This is a versatile vegetable and not only does it taste great, it's full of vitamins, antioxidants, fibre and iodine.

Avocados

Avocados are a source of healthy fats and they are packed with nutrients. It can benefit blood sugar levels, inflammation and reduces metabolic issues. They make a great on-the-go snack as they are neatly packaged and will keep your energy levels balanced.

Coconut Oil

Make coconut oil a store cupboard essential. It's a great food for your thyroid as coconut oil contains medium-chain fatty acids that raise basal body temperature, increase your metabolism and aid weight loss. Avoid hydrogenated oils and margarines completely as they block thyroid function. Your body needs healthy fats and adding coconut oil is a positive step forward.

Fish

Not only is fish rich in omega oils but it also contains zinc and iodine which is essential for thyroid function. However, fish can contain high levels of mercury so only eat seafood which is safe (see foods list). Omega 3 oil is required for healthy brain function, immunity, hormone production, heart health, arthritis and fertility. If you would rather avoid fish you can still get omega 3 oil from olive oil, walnuts, chia seeds, flax seeds and flaxseed oil.

Sea vegetables

Seaweeds such as nori, kombu, wakame, kelp and dulse are a good way to boost you iodine levels and improve thyroid function.

Green Leafy Vegetables

Spinach, Swiss chard and kale are all rich sources of B vitamins which are essential for healthy hormone production and are packed full of amazing antioxidants.

Beans & Pulses

These are a good source of zinc, B vitamins and selenium plus they are rich in iron and light on the digestion so they'll make a useful addition to your diet.

Almonds

Not only are almonds high in protein and fibre, they contain zinc and B vitamins which are extremely useful for thyroid health.

Coriander (Cilantro)

This amazingly fragrant herb is loaded with minerals, vitamins and is a top food for removing and detoxifying heavy metals in the body. It calms the adrenal glands which is great for anyone with adrenal fatigue, stress or blood sugar issues. Add it to salads, smoothies, curries and casseroles or even by the handful if you like – it really is delicious!

Garlic

Garlic is best known for being antibacterial, antiviral and antifungal but it also contains sulphur which helps the detoxification of heavy metals from the liver.

Pectin Rich Fruit

Plums, gooseberries, apples, pears and citrus fruits contain significant amounts of pectin which is so good to aid elimination and detoxify mercury in the body. Don't be afraid to add in as much of the peel into smoothies or when peeling an orange or grapefruit, eat as much of the pith (the creamy coloured layer between the outer peel and flesh) as that is where most of the pectin lies.

Adrenal Fatigue & Blood Sugar Imbalance

Symptoms of adrenal fatigue (also known as adrenal insufficiency) and hypoglycaemia (low blood sugar) often go hand in hand. This is because the adrenal glands regulate adrenaline and not just in response to stress but also blood glucose levels. When blood sugar levels are low the adrenals release more adrenaline which can make you feel anxious and stressed. The knock on effect is that it creates reactions with all the hormones. Eating regularly and avoiding spikes to your blood glucose levels caused be sugar and other stimulants such as cigarettes, alcohol and caffeine is the way forward. Keeping your blood glucose levels balanced and avoiding stress where possible will help your thyroid health.

Is Coffee Giving You A Boost?

Actually, far from giving you a hit of energy, your morning coffee may be doing just the opposite. Coffee is a known stimulant and if you are struggling with an underactive thyroid (or even overactive!) it can be over stimulating for the adrenal glands, causing inflammation, unbalancing your blood sugar and upsetting your hormonal balance. This can result in you feeling even more fatigued and unwell so coffee really is best avoided. Contrary to giving you an energy boost, you may be depleting yourself further.

Do Cruciferous Vegetables Harm The Thyroid?

Certain vegetables such as cauliflower, broccoli, sprouts, kale and swede have been reported to be 'goitergenic' meaning that they have a negative effect on the production of thyroid hormones. However, the quantity of cruciferous vegetables you would need to consume to be harmful are enormous and you'd be unable to eat that amount. Feel free to eat these vegetables in normal portion sizes and you will be packing in those nutrients and importantly those antioxidants which are essential to counteract inflammation in the body.

Getting Started

Eating for thyroid health may be easier than you think! To get started, familiarise yourself with the foods list so that you know what you can and can't eat. It can be really useful to go through your kitchen cupboards and weed out any foods which aren't suitable. This will make it easier for you to find something tasty without being tempted by other foods which may not be helpful.

Read the labels and be realistic about what pre-prepared foods contain, especially when it comes to the sugar in foods. You'd be amazed how much sugar is added to savoury foods and pay special attention to sauces and relishes like sweet chilli sauce and ketchup which mostly consist of sugar. If you would rather just reduce your sugar consumption, make sure you avoid those biscuits, desserts, sweets and cakes which will keep you hooked on sugar and prevent you getting over any sugar cravings you may have.

After a few days it will become so much easier and when you start the feel the benefits you'll be inspired to keep it up.

Cutting out gluten may be the biggest hurdle for some, although if you already know you are coeliac or gluten intolerant, you probably have gluten-free staples in your food supplies.

Keeping it simple is often the best way to get started by using basic fresh ingredients and adding in herbs and/or spices for flavour. Remember if you are used to eating processed foods your taste buds may need to adjust to subtler flavours rather than the whammy of sugar and salt so hang in there! You really can happily eat better and improve your health.

Organic products do tend to be more expensive but if your budget allows it is the best option and you can be sure your health boosting fruits and vegetables won't have pesticides and chemical sprays sabotaging their benefits.

Really load those vegetables and fruits into your diet and you can fill any nutritional deficiencies you might have. You can heap green leafy salads onto the side of your plate and you won't be adding many calories but you will be boosting the goodness of your meals.

To begin with you might get cravings (it will pass!) and diverting yourself is a great tactic to take your mind off it. Going for a walk, taking a relaxing bath or getting some exercise can all help. Remember that exercise produces endorphins which are the 'happy hormones' and will give your mood a boost.

If you're used to medicating yourself with chocolate bars this might be a smaller adjustment than you think. Chocolate itself is good for you it's when it's combined with sugar that's the problem. A square or two of good quality dark chocolate can be enough to satisfy your taste buds although some find it's easier to wait until they feel better before adding in anything too tempting.

You can stock up your kitchen with healthy essentials and check out the recipes for some simple meals or ideas which you can look forward to eating. There really is no better time than now to get started.

Wishing you great health!

Recipes

BREAKFAST

Coconut & Lime Salad Smoothie

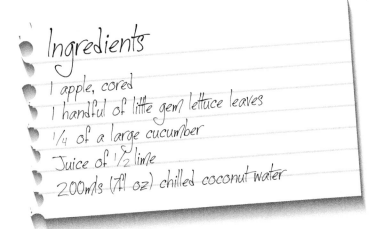

Ingredients

1 apple, cored
1 handful of little gem lettuce leaves
1/4 of a large cucumber
Juice of 1/2 lime
200mls (7fl oz) chilled coconut water

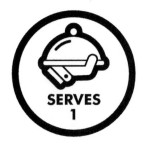

SERVES
1

Method

Place all of the ingredients into a blender and blitz until smooth. Serve straight away.

Tropical Avocado Smoothie

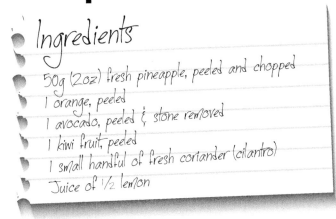

Ingredients

50g (2oz) fresh pineapple, peeled and chopped
1 orange, peeled
1 avocado, peeled & stone removed
1 kiwi fruit, peeled
1 small handful of fresh coriander (cilantro)
Juice of 1/2 lemon

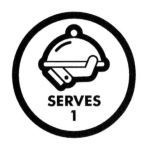

SERVES
1

Method

Place all of the ingredients into a blender and add enough water to cover them. Process until creamy and smooth.

Orange, Celery & Ginger Smoothie

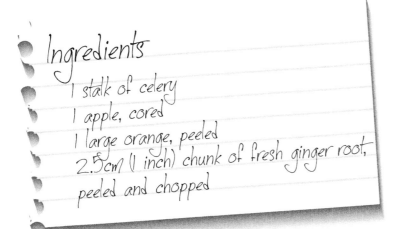

Ingredients

1 stalk of celery
1 apple, cored
1 large orange, peeled
2.5cm (1 inch) chunk of fresh ginger root,
peeled and chopped

SERVES
1

Method

Put all the ingredients into a blender with some water and blitz until smooth. Add ice to make your smoothie really refreshing.

Berry Cocktail

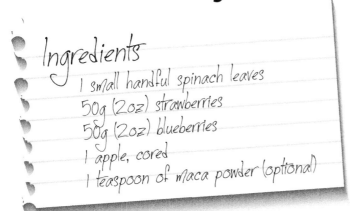

Ingredients

1 small handful spinach leaves
50g (2oz) strawberries
50g (2oz) blueberries
1 apple, cored
1 teaspoon of maca powder (optional)

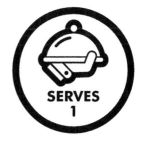

SERVES
1

Method

Place the ingredients into a blender and add just enough water to cover the ingredients. Process until smooth.

Grapefruit & Carrot Refresher

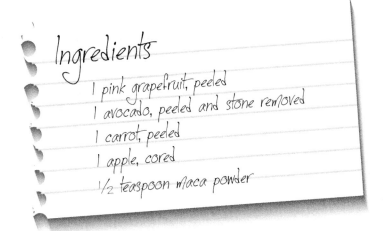

Ingredients

1 pink grapefruit, peeled
1 avocado, peeled and stone removed
1 carrot, peeled
1 apple, cored
1/2 teaspoon maca powder

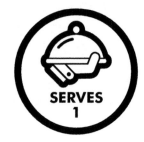

SERVES
1

Method

Place all the ingredients into a blender with enough water to cover them and blitz until smooth.

Sweet Cherry Crush

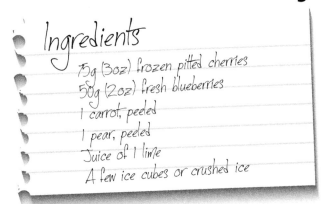

Ingredients

75g (3oz) frozen pitted cherries
50g (2oz) fresh blueberries
1 carrot, peeled
1 pear, peeled
Juice of 1 lime
A few ice cubes or crushed ice

SERVES
1

Method

Place all of the ingredients into a blender with enough water to cover them and process until smooth.

Golden Banana & Mango Delight

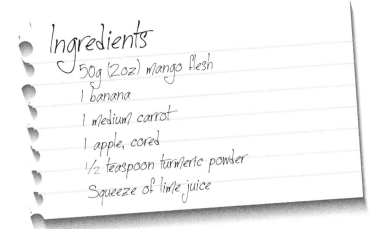

Ingredients
- 50g (2oz) mango flesh
- 1 banana
- 1 medium carrot
- 1 apple, cored
- 1/2 teaspoon turmeric powder
- Squeeze of lime juice

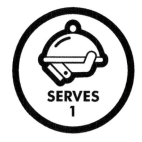

SERVES
1

Method

Place all the ingredients into a blender with just enough water to cover them. Process until smooth.

Creamy Peach Smoothie

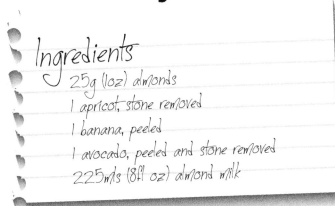

Ingredients
- 25g (1oz) almonds
- 1 apricot, stone removed
- 1 banana, peeled
- 1 avocado, peeled and stone removed
- 225mls (8fl oz) almond milk

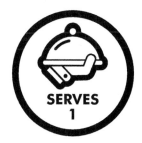

SERVES
1

Method

Place all of the ingredients into a blender and process until smooth. Serve and drink straight away.

Sweet Superfood Juice

Ingredients

2 celery stalks
1 large kale leaf
1 cucumber
1 pear, cored
1 apple, cored

1 lemon
1 small handful of fresh coriander (cilantro)
2cm (1 inch) chunk of ginger, peeled

SERVES
1

Method

Process all of the ingredients through a juicer and pour the juice into a glass. Add a few ice cubes and drink straight away.

Melon & Raspberry Smoothie

Ingredients

25g (1oz) frozen raspberries
6 cherries, de-stoned
1 apple, cored
1/2 cantaloupe melon, flesh only

SERVES
1

Method

Place all the ingredients into a blender and add just enough water to cover the ingredients. Blitz until smooth. Serve and drink straight away.

Strawberry & Avocado Smoothie

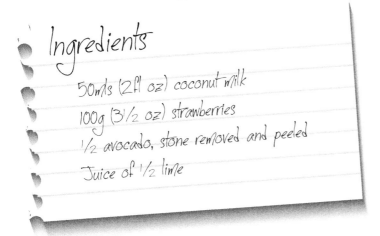

Ingredients

50mls (2fl oz) coconut milk

100g (3½ oz) strawberries

½ avocado, stone removed and peeled

Juice of ½ lime

SERVES 1

Method

Toss all of the ingredients into a blender. Blitz until creamy. If it seems too thick you can add some water. Pour and enjoy!

Apple & Celery Smoothie

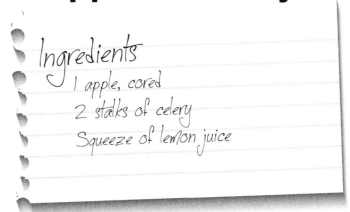

Ingredients

1 apple, cored

2 stalks of celery

Squeeze of lemon juice

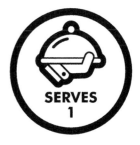

SERVES 1

Method

Place all the ingredients into a food processor and cover them with a little water. Blitz until smooth.

Coriander Scramble

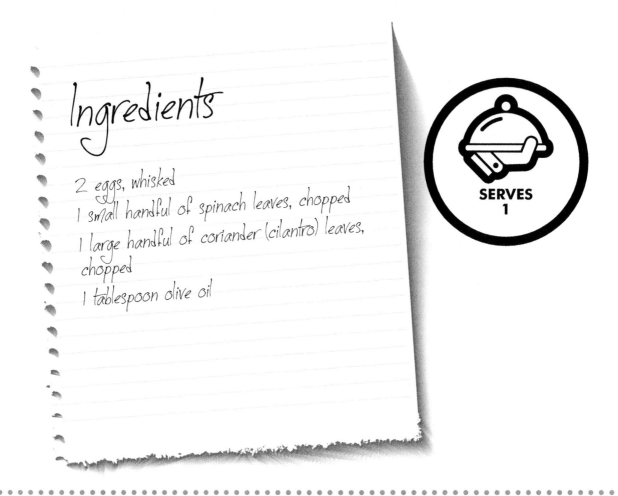

Ingredients

2 eggs, whisked
1 small handful of spinach leaves, chopped
1 large handful of coriander (cilantro) leaves, chopped
1 tablespoon olive oil

**SERVES
1**

Method

Whisk the eggs in a bowl and add in the spinach and coriander (cilantro). Heat the oil in a frying pan, pour into the egg mixture and using a spatula, move the eggs around the pan until they are set. Serve and eat straight away.

Herby Tomato Frittata

Ingredients

75g (3oz) pitted black olives, halved

10 ripe cherry tomatoes, halved

4 large eggs

2 slices of cooked ham, chopped

1 handful of fresh coriander (cilantro), chopped

1 small handful of fresh chives, chopped

1 tablespoon olive oil

SERVES 2

Method

Break the eggs into a bowl and whisk them then add in the coriander (cilantro), chives, ham, olives and tomatoes. Heat the oil in a small frying pan and pour in the egg mixture. Cook until the egg mixture completely sets. Place the frittata under a hot grill for 3 minutes to finish it off. Carefully remove it from the pan. Cut into slices and serve.

Mushroom & Tomato Omelette

**SERVES
1**

Ingredients

2 eggs, beaten

100g (3½ oz) mushrooms, chopped

1 handful spinach

1 tomato, cut into slices

1 tablespoon fresh coriander (cilantro), chopped

1 tablespoon olive oil

Method

Heat the olive oil in a saucepan, add the mushrooms, tomato and spinach and cook until softened. Remove them and set aside. Pour the beaten eggs into the frying pan, spoon the vegetable mixture over the top and sprinkle on the coriander (cilantro). When the eggs have set, serve the omelette onto a plate. Eat straight away.

Baked Egg Avocados

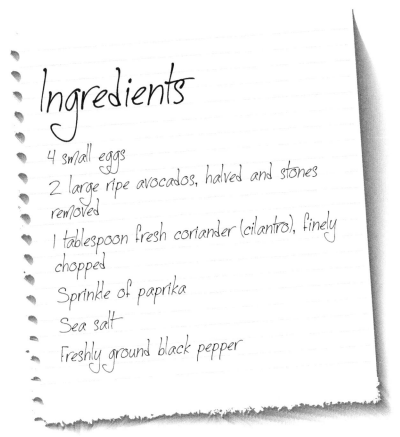

Ingredients

4 small eggs

2 large ripe avocados, halved and stones removed

1 tablespoon fresh coriander (cilantro), finely chopped

Sprinkle of paprika

Sea salt

Freshly ground black pepper

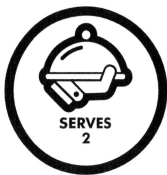

SERVES 2

Method

Place half of an avocado in a ramekin dish with the hollow facing upwards. Crack an egg into the hollow of each avocado, although you may need to remove a little avocado flesh to do so. Sprinkle with coriander (cilantro), salt and pepper. Bake in an oven, preheated to 220C/440F and cook for 20 minutes until the eggs have set. Serve immediately.

LUNCH

Lemon Poached Salmon & Capers

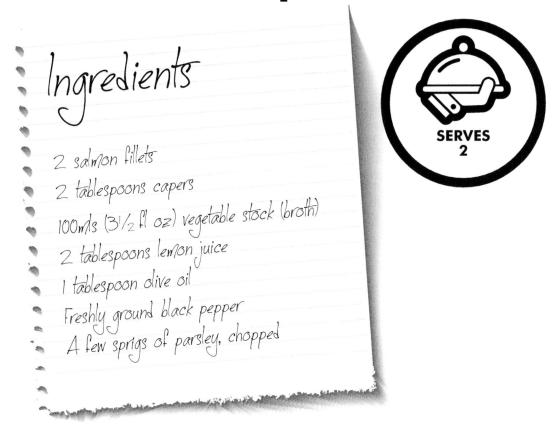

Ingredients

- 2 salmon fillets
- 2 tablespoons capers
- 100mls (3½ fl oz) vegetable stock (broth)
- 2 tablespoons lemon juice
- 1 tablespoon olive oil
- Freshly ground black pepper
- A few sprigs of parsley, chopped

SERVES 2

Method

Heat the stock (broth) and lemon juice in a frying pan, gently place the salmon into the pan, reduce the heat and simmer until the salmon is completely cooked and opaque, easily flaking away. Remove the salmon, cover it and keep it warm. Turn up the heat on the frying pan and reduce the remaining stock until it is around half. Add in the oil, capers and pepper. Serve the fish with a drizzle of the sauce. Scatter some parsley over the top.

Mildy Spiced Bean Balls

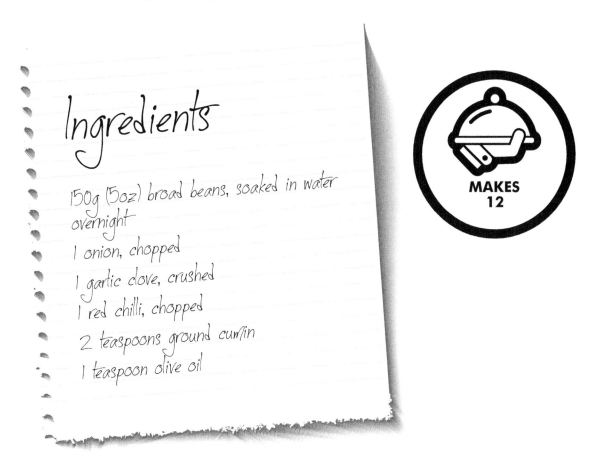

Ingredients

150g (5oz) broad beans, soaked in water overnight

1 onion, chopped

1 garlic clove, crushed

1 red chilli, chopped

2 teaspoons ground cumin

1 teaspoon olive oil

MAKES 12

Method

Place all of the ingredients into a food processor and blend to a smooth paste. Shape the mixture into balls and place them on a greased baking tray. Transfer them to the oven and bake at 180/360F for 20 minutes.

King Prawn & Garlicky Spinach

SERVES 4

Ingredients

450g (1lb) king prawns (shrimps), shelled

200g (7oz) spinach leaves, washed

4 tomatoes, chopped

4 spring onions (scallions), chopped

3 cloves of garlic, crushed

2 tablespoons olive oil

Method

Heat the oil in a frying pan, add the tomatoes, 1 clove of garlic, spring onions (scallions) and cook for 4-5 minutes. Add the prawns (shrimps) and cook until they are pink throughout. Remove them and set them aside. Add the spinach and the remaining garlic to the pan and cook until the spinach has wilted. You can add a little hot water or oil to the pan if you need extra moisture. Serve the spinach onto plates and add the prawn mixture on top. Serve and eat straight away.

Courgette 'Spaghetti' With Avocado & Pine Nuts

**SERVES
1**

Ingredients

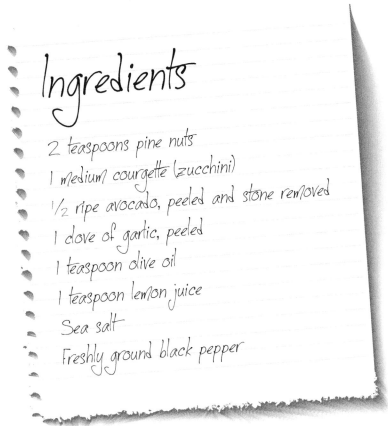

2 teaspoons pine nuts

1 medium courgette (zucchini)

½ ripe avocado, peeled and stone removed

1 clove of garlic, peeled

1 teaspoon olive oil

1 teaspoon lemon juice

Sea salt

Freshly ground black pepper

Method

Use a spiraliser or if you don't have one, use a vegetable peeler and cut the courgette (zucchini) into thin strips. Heat a teaspoon of oil in a frying pan, add the courgette (zucchini) and cook for 4-5 minutes or until it has softened. In the meantime, place the avocado, garlic and lemon juice and a teaspoon of olive oil into a blender and process until smooth. Add the avocado mixture to the courgette (zucchini) and stir it well. Season with salt and pepper. Serve and sprinkle with pine nuts.

Sundried Tomato Chicken & Mushrooms

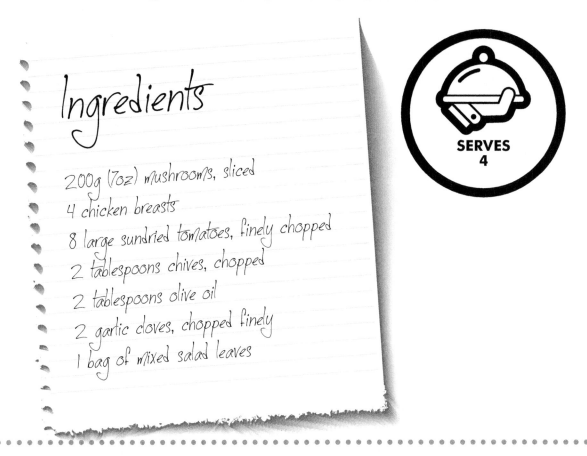

SERVES 4

Ingredients

200g (7oz) mushrooms, sliced

4 chicken breasts

8 large sundried tomatoes, finely chopped

2 tablespoons chives, chopped

2 tablespoons olive oil

2 garlic cloves, chopped finely

1 bag of mixed salad leaves

Method

Place the tomatoes into a bowl and add the chives and garlic. Mix well. Make a horizontal incision in each of the chicken breasts and press some of the tomato mixture into them. Heat the oil in a frying pan and add the chicken. Cook for around 6 minutes on each side. Add in the mushrooms towards the end of cooking and cook until they have softened. Scatter some mixed salad leaves onto plates and serve the chicken and mushrooms. Eat straight away.

Mango Salsa

Ingredients

4 ripe tomatoes, diced
3 cloves garlic, finely chopped
1 red onion, chopped
1 green chilli, de-seeded and finely chopped
1 bunch fresh coriander (cilantro), chopped
1 mango, stone removed, peeled and diced
1 avocado, stone removed, peeled and diced
Juice of ½ fresh lime juice
3 tablespoons olive oil

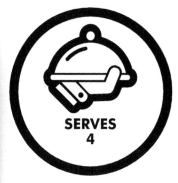

**SERVES
4**

Method

Combine the mango, avocado, tomatoes, chilli, coriander (cilantro) and garlic in a bowl. Mix in the lime juice, onion and olive oil. Chill before serving.

Tomato & Olive Salad

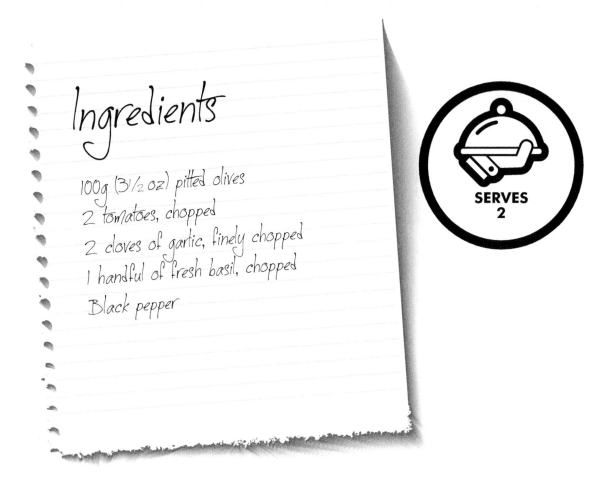

Ingredients

100g (3½ oz) pitted olives
2 tomatoes, chopped
2 cloves of garlic, finely chopped
1 handful of fresh basil, chopped
Black pepper

SERVES
2

Method

Place all of the ingredients into a bowl and toss them together. Serve and enjoy.

Broad Bean Salad

Ingredients

450g (1lb) frozen broad beans, cooked according to instructions
2 ripe tomatoes, chopped
2 cloves garlic, crushed
1 small red onion, finely chopped
1 cucumber, diced
1 teaspoon ground cumin
Small bunch of fresh basil
Small bunch of fresh coriander (cilantro), chopped
Juice of 1 lemon
3 tablespoons olive oil
Sea salt
Freshly ground black pepper

SERVES 4

Method

Combine cooked broad beans, tomatoes, onion and cucumber in a salad bowl. Stir in the basil, coriander (cilantro), garlic, cumin, parsley, lemon juice and olive oil. Season with salt and pepper to taste. Serve and enjoy.

Stuffed Tomatoes

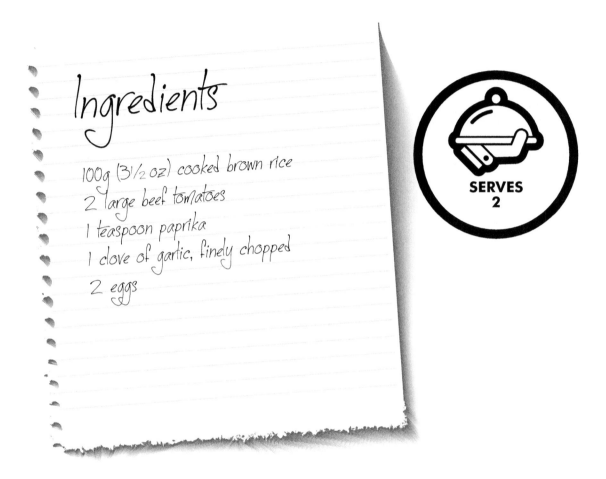

Ingredients

100g (3½ oz) cooked brown rice
2 large beef tomatoes
1 teaspoon paprika
1 clove of garlic, finely chopped
2 eggs

SERVES 2

Method

Cut and remove the very top of the tomato to expose the seeds inside. Scoop out the seeds and discard them. Stand the tomatoes upright for 5 minutes to let any moisture drain out. In a bowl combine the rice, garlic and paprika. Spoon the mixture into the tomatoes. Break an egg into the top of each tomato. Place them on a baking sheet and cook them in the oven, preheated to 180C/ 360F and cook them for about 20 minutes or until the eggs are completely set. Serve and eat straight away.

Sweetcorn &
Black Bean Salad

Ingredients

- 225g (8oz) sweetcorn
- 2 x 400g (14oz) tins of black beans, drained and rinsed
- 6 spring onions (scallions), thinly sliced
- 2 tomatoes, chopped
- 2 tablespoons fresh coriander (cilantro) chopped
- 1 clove garlic, minced
- 1 teaspoon sea salt
- 1 avocado, stone removed, peeled and diced
- 1 red pepper (bell pepper), chopped
- 1/2 teaspoon chilli powder (optional)
- 6 tablespoons olive oil
- Juice of 1 lime

SERVES
4

Method

Place the lime juice, olive oil, garlic, salt and chilli in a bowl and mix well. In a large serving bowl, combine the beans, sweetcorn, avocado, pepper, tomatoes, spring onions (scallions) and coriander (cilantro). Pour the oil mixture over the salad ingredients and mix well. Chill before serving.

Leek & Potato Soup

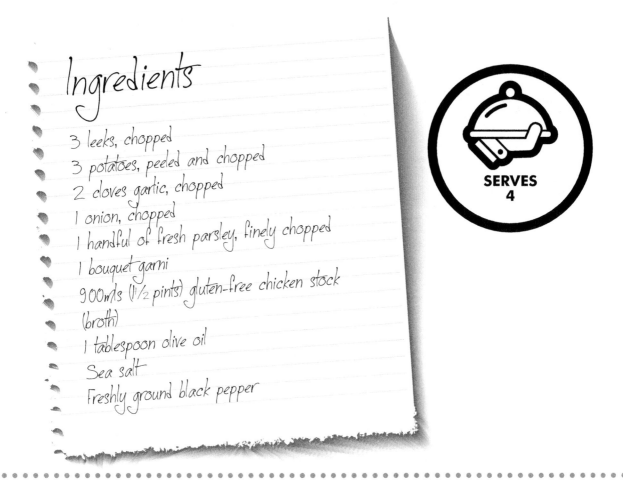

Ingredients

3 leeks, chopped
3 potatoes, peeled and chopped
2 cloves garlic, chopped
1 onion, chopped
1 handful of fresh parsley, finely chopped
1 bouquet garni
900mls (1½ pints) gluten-free chicken stock (broth)
1 tablespoon olive oil
Sea salt
Freshly ground black pepper

SERVES 4

Method

Heat the oil in a saucepan, add the onion and cook until they have softened. Add in the leeks, garlic, potatoes and cook for around 2 minutes. Add the stock (broth), bouquet garni and season with salt and pepper. Bring it to the boil, reduce the heat and simmer for 30 minutes. Remove the bouquet garni and discard it. Using a hand blender or food processor, blitz the soup until smooth and creamy. Stir in the parsley and serve.

Thai Style Squash Soup

Ingredients

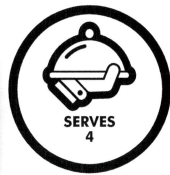

SERVES 4

5cm (2.5inch) chunk of root ginger, peeled and finely

2 teaspoons curry powder (or Thai curry paste)

1 butternut squash, peeled, de-seeded and chopped

1 large onion, chopped

1 tablespoon fresh coriander (cilantro)

900mls (1½ pints) gluten-free vegetable stock

125mls (4fl oz) coconut milk

1 tablespoon olive oil

Method

Heat the oil in a saucepan, add the onion and cook until it softens. Add the squash, curry powder (or paste), ginger and vegetable stock (broth). Bring the soup to the boil, reduce the heat and simmer for 20 minutes or until the squash is soft. Using a hand blender or a food processor, blitz the soup until smooth. It's advisable to let it cool slightly before transferring it to a food processor. Stir in the coconut milk and warm the soup completely. Serve into bowls with a sprinkling of coriander (cilantro).

45

Butternut Squash & Orange Soup

**SERVES
4**

Ingredients

- 450g (1lb) butternut squash, peeled, de-seeded and chopped
- 3 tablespoons fresh coriander (cilantro)
- 1 onion, chopped
- 1 teaspoon ground coriander (cilantro)
- 1 tablespoon olive oil
- 1200mls (2 pints) hot water
- Grated zest and juice of 1 orange

Method

Heat the oil in a saucepan, add the onion and cook for 5 minutes. Add in the squash and cook for 5 minutes. Stir in the ground coriander (cilantro), orange zest and hot water. Reduce the heat and simmer for 10 minutes. Stir in the coriander (cilantro) and orange juice. Using a hand blender or food processor blend the soup until smooth. Re-heat if necessary before serving. Serve with a sprinkling of parsley.

Gazpacho

Ingredients

10 tomatoes, de-seeded and chopped

2 red peppers (bell peppers), de-seeded and chopped

4 cloves of garlic, chopped

2 medium cucumbers, peeled and chopped

1 teaspoon chilli flakes

4 teaspoons olive oil

4 tablespoons apple cider vinegar

Sea salt

Freshly ground black pepper

**SERVES
4**

Method

Heat the oil in a saucepan, add the onion and cook until it softens. Add the squash, curry powder (or paste), ginger and vegetable stock (broth). Bring the soup to the boil, reduce the heat and simmer for 20 minutes or until the squash is soft. Using a hand blender or a food processor, blitz the soup until smooth. It's advisable to let it cool slightly before transferring it to a food processor. Stir in the coconut milk and warm the soup completely. Serve into bowls with a sprinkling of coriander (cilantro).

Quick Carrot & Coriander Soup

SERVES 2

Ingredients

5 medium carrots, peeled and chopped

1 onion, peeled and chopped

1 teaspoon ground coriander (cilantro)

1 tablespoon of olive oil

A large handful of fresh coriander (cilantro)

Sea salt

Freshly ground black pepper

900mls (1½ pints) gluten-free vegetable stock (broth)

Fresh coriander (cilantro) for garnish

Method

Heat the oil in a saucepan, add the carrots and onion and cook for around 5 minutes until they have softened. Add in the stock (broth), ground and fresh coriander (cilantro) and bring it to the boil. Continue cooking for 10 minutes. Using a hand blender or food processor, blitz the soup until smooth and creamy. Season with salt and pepper. Serve into bowls and garnish with a little fresh coriander.

Tomato & Lentil Soup

SERVES 4

Ingredients

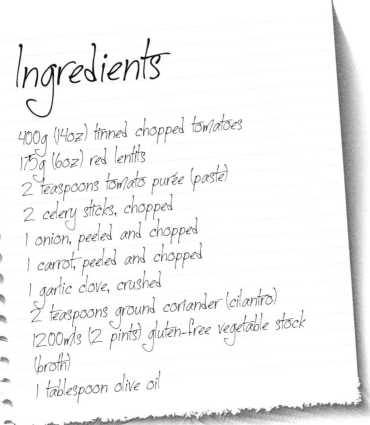

400g (14oz) tinned chopped tomatoes

175g (6oz) red lentils

2 teaspoons tomato purée (paste)

2 celery sticks, chopped

1 onion, peeled and chopped

1 carrot, peeled and chopped

1 garlic clove, crushed

2 teaspoons ground coriander (cilantro)

1200mls (2 pints) gluten-free vegetable stock (broth)

1 tablespoon olive oil

Method

Heat the oil in a saucepan, add the onion and cook until the onion softens. Add in the celery and carrot, garlic and coriander (cilantro) and cook for a further minute. Add in the stock (broth), lentils, tomatoes and tomato purée (paste) and cook for 20-30 |minutes. Using a hand blender or food processor blend the soup until smooth. Serve and enjoy.

49

Celeriac & Pear Soup

Ingredients

2 pears, cored, peeled and chopped

1 head of celeriac, peeled and chopped

1 onion, chopped

1 teaspoon ground coriander (cilantro)

2.5cm (1 inch) chunk fresh root ginger

600mls (1 pint) gluten-free vegetable stock (broth)

2 tablespoons olive oil

Freshly ground black pepper

SERVES 6

Method

Heat the oil in a large saucepan, add the onion, celeriac and ginger and cook for 5 minutes. Pour in the vegetable stock (broth) and add the pear, and coriander (cilantro). Bring it to the boil, reduce the heat and simmer for 20-25 minutes. Using a hand blender or food processor, blend the soup until it's smooth. You can add extra stock (broth) or hot water to make the soup thinner if you wish. Season with pepper then serve into bowls.

Sweet Potato Fries

Ingredients

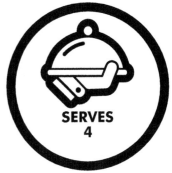

4 large sweet potatoes, peeled and cut into strips 1-2cm in thickness

2 tablespoons olive oil

1 teaspoon rosemary (fresh or dried), finely chopped

Sea salt

Freshly ground black pepper

Method

In a large bowl, coat the sweet potato strips in the olive oil and rosemary and season with salt and pepper. Line a large backing tray with parchment paper. Spread the sweet potatoes over the tray in a single layer and if you need to, use a second tray. Preheat the oven to 220C/440F and bake the sweet potatoes for 20 minutes or until completely cooked and slightly golden.

Baked Olives

Ingredients

250g (9oz) whole mixed olives, drained
2 tablespoons apple cider vinegar
1 tablespoons fresh orange juice
1 tablespoons olive oil
2 cloves garlic, finely chopped
2 sprigs fresh rosemary
1 tablespoon fresh parsley, chopped
1 tablespoon chopped fresh oregano
2 teaspoons grated orange zest
Pinch of chilli flakes

**SERVES
6**

Method

Preheat the oven to 190C/ 380F. Place the olives in an ovenproof dish and mix in the vinegar, orange juice, olive oil, rosemary and garlic. Transfer them to the oven and cook for 15 minutes. Remove the rosemary and add in the herbs, chilli flakes and orange zest. Can be served warm or cold.

Gluten Free Garlic
& Herb Crackers

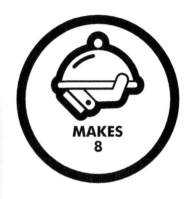

**MAKES
8**

Ingredients

75g (3oz) chia seeds

75g (3oz) sunflower seeds

50g (2oz) ground almonds (almond meal/
almond flour)

2 teaspoons herbs de Provence or mixed
herbs

1 clove of garlic, crushed

1/2 teaspoon sea salt

250mls (8fl oz) cold water

Method

In a bowl, combine the sunflower seeds, chia seeds, almonds, garlic, herbs and salt. Pour in the water and mix really well until the ingredients thicken. Grease and line a baking tray and spoon the mixture into it, spreading and smoothing it out. Transfer it to the oven, preheated to 170C/340F and cook for 25 minutes. Remove it and carefully cut it into slices. Return it to the oven and cook for another 25 minutes. Once cooled, store in an airtight container. Use as a snack or serve with salads and dips.

Sweet Potato Cakes

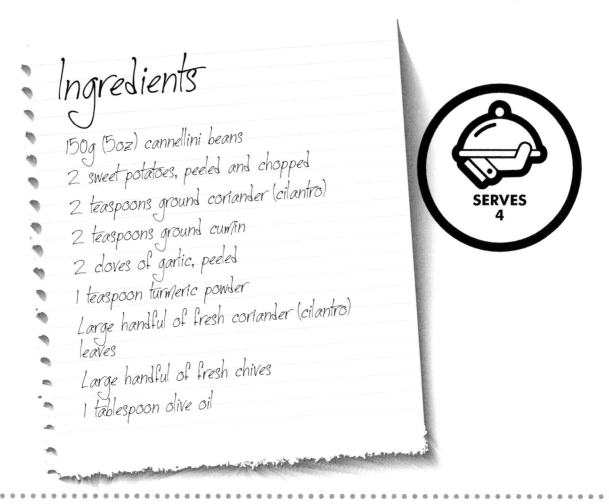

Ingredients

150g (5oz) cannellini beans

2 sweet potatoes, peeled and chopped

2 teaspoons ground coriander (cilantro)

2 teaspoons ground cumin

2 cloves of garlic, peeled

1 teaspoon turmeric powder

Large handful of fresh coriander (cilantro) leaves

Large handful of fresh chives

1 tablespoon olive oil

SERVES 4

Method

Steam the sweet potatoes until soft and tender. Set it aside until it cools down. Place all of the ingredients, apart from the olive oil, into a food processor and blitz until you have everything is completely soft and combined. Shape the mixture into balls then press them flat. Store them in the fridge for an hour to become firm. Grease a baking tray with the olive oil. Place the sweet potato cakes onto the tray and bake in the oven at 220C/440F for around 15 minutes or until slightly golden.

Pinto Bean, Lime & Coriander Salad

Ingredients

400g (14oz) tin of pinto beans, rinsed and drained

250g (9oz) cooked brown rice, cooled

2 large handfuls of fresh coriander (cilantro)

3 spring onions (scallions) finely chopped

1 tablespoon olive oil

Juice of 1 lime

Sea salt

Freshly ground black pepper

SERVES 2

Method

Place the beans, rice, coriander (cilantro), spring onions (scallions), olive oil and lime juice into a bowl and mix well. Season with salt and pepper. Chill before serving.

Spicy Black Bean Hummus

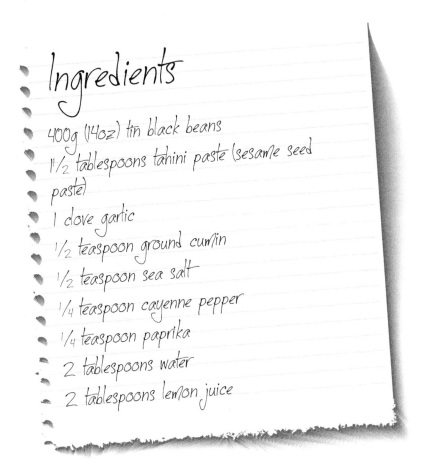

Ingredients

400g (14oz) tin black beans

1½ tablespoons tahini paste (sesame seed paste)

1 clove garlic

½ teaspoon ground cumin

½ teaspoon sea salt

¼ teaspoon cayenne pepper

¼ teaspoon paprika

2 tablespoons water

2 tablespoons lemon juice

Method

Place all of the ingredients and process until smooth. Serve as a dip for vegetable crudités or use with salads.

Lemon Hummus With Celery

SERVES 4

Ingredients

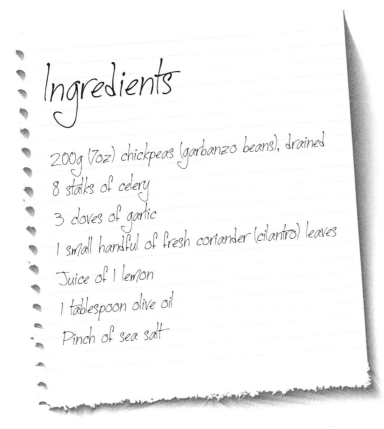

200g (7oz) chickpeas (garbanzo beans), drained

8 stalks of celery

3 cloves of garlic

1 small handful of fresh coriander (cilantro) leaves

Juice of 1 lemon

1 tablespoon olive oil

Pinch of sea salt

Method

Place the chickpeas (garbanzo beans), garlic, coriander (cilantro), salt, lemon and oil into a food processor and blitz until smooth. Spoon it into a serving bowl and use as a dip for the celery stalks.

Falafels

Ingredients

400g (14oz) tinned chickpeas (garbanzo beans), drained and rinsed

2 teaspoons ground cumin

1 egg, beaten

1 small onion, finely chopped

1 clove of garlic, crushed

1 teaspoon mixed herbs

Grated zest of 1 lemon

2 tablespoons olive oil

Sea salt

Freshly ground black pepper

SERVES 4

Method

Heat 1 tablespoon of oil in a frying pan, add the onion and garlic and cook gently until they have softened. Place the chickpeas (garbanzo beans), onion and garlic into a bowl and mash them until they are completely soft. Alternatively you could use a food processor. Add in the herbs, lemon zest, cumin, egg and mix well. Season with salt and pepper. Using clean hands, roll the mixture into small balls and lay them onto a baking tray. Cover them and place them in the fridge for around 30 minutes, to firm up. Preheat the oven to 200C/400F. Brush the falafels with a tablespoon of olive oil and place the tray into the oven. Cook for 20-25 minutes or until they are golden. Allow them to cool before serving. Serve with a hummus dip or use as an addition to salads.

DINNER

Jambalaya

Ingredients

400g (14oz) tin of chopped tomatoes
400g (14oz) rice
200g (7oz) skinless salmon fillet, diced
100g (3½ oz) large peeled prawns (shrimps)
3 garlic cloves, crushed
2 celery sticks, sliced
1 onion, chopped
1 red pepper (bell pepper), chopped
1 teaspoon mild chilli powder
½ teaspoon ground ginger
½ teaspoon cayenne pepper
A handful of fresh parsley, chopped
900mls (1½ pints) gluten-free vegetable stock (broth)
1½ tablespoon olive oil
Salt and pepper

SERVES 4

Method

Heat the oil in a large saucepan, add the onion and celery and cook, stirring, for about 3 minutes. Add the pepper (bell pepper), garlic, ginger, cayenne, chilli powder and rice, and cook, stirring, for 3 minutes. Add in the stock (broth), reduce the heat, cover and cook for 15 minutes. Add in the tomatoes, prawns (shrimps) and salmon and cook for 4-5 minutes when the salmon and prawns should be completely cooked and pink throughout and the rice is soft. Stir in the parsley. Season with salt and pepper. Serve and enjoy.

Smokey Bean Casserole

Ingredients

- 400g (14oz) pinto beans, drained and rinsed
- 400g (14oz) haricot beans, drained and rinsed
- 400g (14oz) tinned tomatoes, chopped
- 225g (8oz) button mushrooms, halved
- 2 garlic cloves, chopped
- 1 onion, chopped
- 1 small leek, finely chopped
- 1 tablespoon smoked paprika
- 1 red chilli, finely chopped
- 1 large handful of coriander (cilantro) or parsley
- 250mls (8fl oz) gluten-free vegetable stock (broth)
- 1 tablespoon olive oil

SERVES 4

Method

Heat the oil in a saucepan, add the onions and garlic and cook until the onions have softened. Stir in the mushrooms, leeks, chilli, haricot beans, pinto beans, tomatoes and paprika and cook for 5 minutes. Pour in the stock (broth) and simmer for 15 minutes. Stir in the fresh herbs and eat straight away.

Vegetable Bake

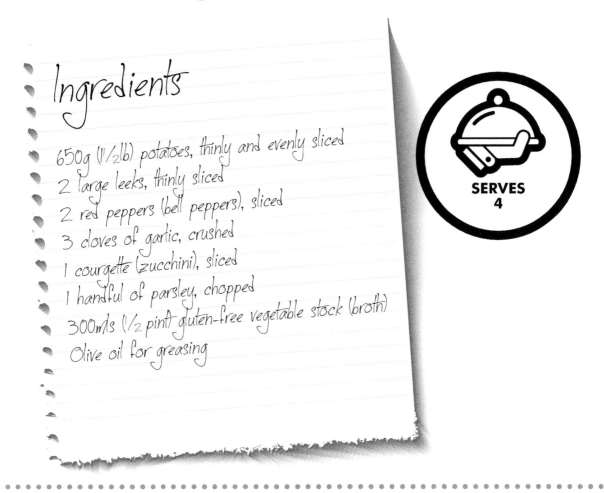

Ingredients

650g (1½lb) potatoes, thinly and evenly sliced
2 large leeks, thinly sliced
2 red peppers (bell peppers), sliced
3 cloves of garlic, crushed
1 courgette (zucchini), sliced
1 handful of parsley, chopped
300mls (½ pint) gluten-free vegetable stock (broth)
Olive oil for greasing

SERVES 4

Method

Grease a large casserole dish with olive oil. Place a layer of potatoes on the bottom of the casserole dish and sprinkle a little parsley on top. Add a layer of leeks, followed by a layer of courgette (zucchini), peppers (bell peppers), garlic and parsley. Place a layer of potatoes on top and repeat until all the vegetables have been used up. Pour on the vegetable stock (broth). Bake in the oven at 180C/360F for 90 minutes until the top is golden.

Citrus Wild Rice & Cannellini Salad

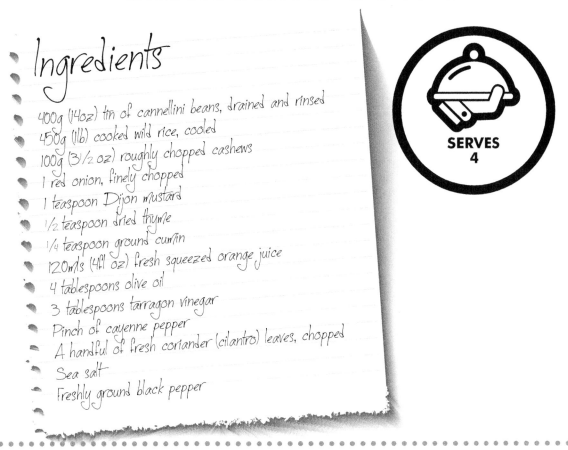

Ingredients

- 400g (14oz) tin of cannellini beans, drained and rinsed
- 450g (1lb) cooked wild rice, cooled
- 100g (3½ oz) roughly chopped cashews
- 1 red onion, finely chopped
- 1 teaspoon Dijon mustard
- ½ teaspoon dried thyme
- ¼ teaspoon ground cumin
- 120mls (4fl oz) fresh squeezed orange juice
- 4 tablespoons olive oil
- 3 tablespoons tarragon vinegar
- Pinch of cayenne pepper
- A handful of fresh coriander (cilantro) leaves, chopped
- Sea salt
- Freshly ground black pepper

SERVES 4

Method

Pour the orange juice, olive oil and vinegar into a cup and stir in the mustard, cumin, cayenne pepper and thyme. Place the onion, coriander (cilantro), cannellini beans, rice and cashews in a bowl and stir in the dressing. Season with salt and pepper. Chill before serving.

Roast Salmon & Asparagus

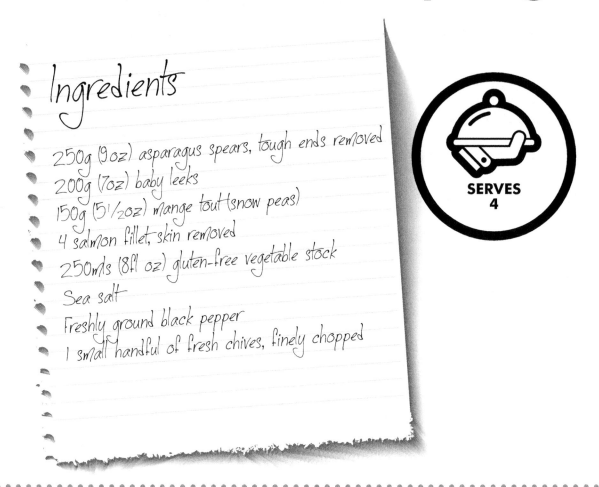

Ingredients

250g (9oz) asparagus spears, tough ends removed
200g (7oz) baby leeks
150g (5½oz) mange tout (snow peas)
4 salmon fillet, skin removed
250mls (8fl oz) gluten-free vegetable stock
Sea salt
Freshly ground black pepper
1 small handful of fresh chives, finely chopped

SERVES 4

Method

Place the leeks, asparagus and mange tout (snow peas) into an ovenproof dish and lay the salmon fillets on top. Pour in the stock (broth) and season with salt and pepper. Transfer it to an oven, preheated to 450F and cook for 13-15 minutes. The salmon should be opaque, pink and cooked through. Serve with a sprinkling of fresh chives.

Steak & Root Vegetable Casserole

Ingredients

- 675g (1 ½ lb) stewing steak
- 175g (6oz) button mushrooms
- 8 shallots, peeled
- 2 carrots, peeled and chopped
- 1 parsnip, peeled and chopped
- 1 tablespoons olive oil
- 1-2 teaspoons dried mixed herbs
- Sea salt
- Freshly ground black pepper
- 600mls (1 pint) gluten-free beef stock (broth)

SERVES 4

Method

Heat a tablespoon of olive oil in a pan, add the steak and brown it on all sides. Transfer the steak to an ovenproof dish. Add in the mushrooms, shallots, carrots, parsnip, herbs and stock (broth). Place a lid on the dish or cover it with foil. Transfer it to the oven and cook at 150C/300F for 1 ½ to 2 hours and the meat should be tender. Season with salt and pepper. Serve with new potatoes or squash mash.

Lamb & Mint Quinoa

Ingredients

- 450g (1lb) lean lamb steaks
- 225g (8oz) asparagus, roughly chopped
- 225g (8oz) frozen peas
- 200g (7oz) mange tout (snow peas)
- 150g (5oz) quinoa
- 2 tablespoons fresh mint, roughly chopped
- 1 garlic clove, crushed
- Juice of 1 lemon
- 1 tablespoon olive oil
- 2 teaspoons olive oil
- Chopped mint for garnish

SERVES 4

Method

In a bowl, combine a teaspoon of olive oil, lemon juice and garlic in a bowl. Add the lamb, coat it in the mixture and marinate it for around 30 minutes. In the meantime, cook the quinoa according to the instructions, usually for around 15-20 minutes, until fluffy. Add the mint to the quinoa and stir. Heat a teaspoon of oil in a frying pan; add the lamb and cook for 9-10 minutes or until it's done to your liking. While the lamb is cooking, steam the asparagus, peas and mange tout (snow peas) for around 4 minutes until they are tender. Place the vegetables into a bowl and stir in the lemon juice, garlic and a tablespoon of olive oil and a few chopped mint leaves. Add in the quinoa and mix well. Serve the quinoa salad with the lamb on top.

Tomato & Chilli 'Rice'

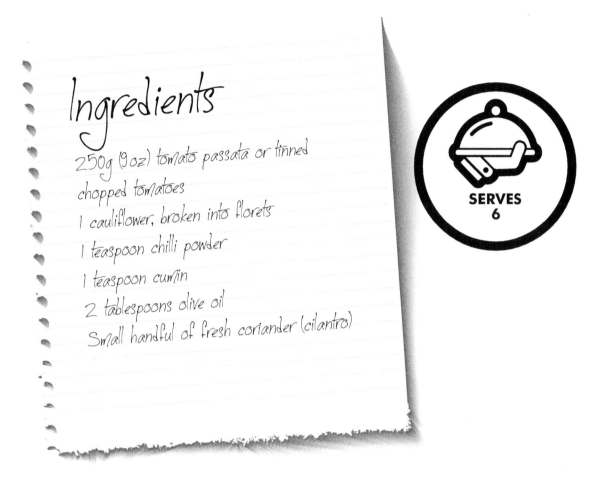

Ingredients

250g (9oz) tomato passata or tinned chopped tomatoes

1 cauliflower, broken into florets

1 teaspoon chilli powder

1 teaspoon cumin

2 tablespoons olive oil

Small handful of fresh coriander (cilantro)

SERVES 6

Method

Place the cauliflower into a food processor and blitz until fine and rice-like. Heat the olive oil in a large frying pan, add the cauliflower and cook for 5-7 minutes or until the vegetables have softened Add the tomato, chilli, passata/chopped tomatoes and cumin and warm it through. Sprinkle in the coriander (cilantro) just before serving.

Spanish Roast Mackerel

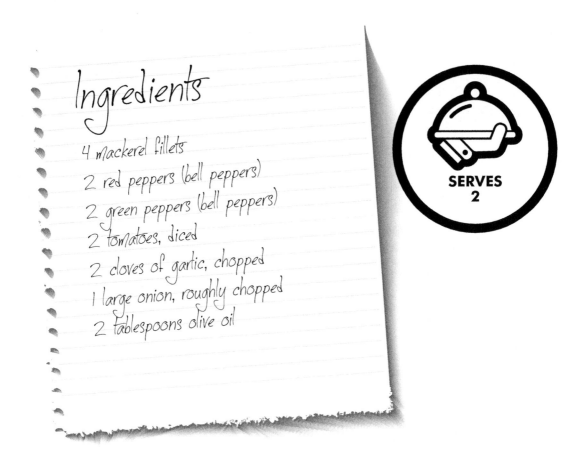

Ingredients

4 mackerel fillets
2 red peppers (bell peppers)
2 green peppers (bell peppers)
2 tomatoes, diced
2 cloves of garlic, chopped
1 large onion, roughly chopped
2 tablespoons olive oil

SERVES 2

Method

Place the whole peppers, tomatoes, onion and garlic into an ovenproof dish and coat them in olive oil. Transfer them to an oven, preheated to 200C/400F and cook for around 35 minutes. Remove them from the oven and place the peppers into a plastic zip lock bag or cover them with cling film. In the meantime, place the mackerel onto a baking tray and cook them in the oven for 10 minutes or until they are completely cooked. Remove the peppers from the bag and slice them roughly, removing the seeds. Place the tomatoes, onion, garlic and mackerel into a bowl and combine. Can be served warm or cold.

Lentil Curry

Ingredients

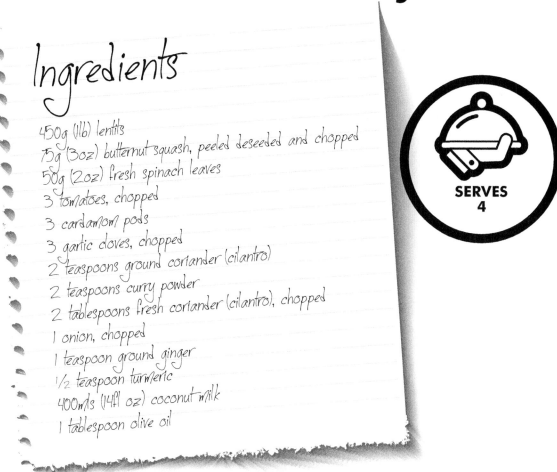

450g (1lb) lentils
75g (3oz) butternut squash, peeled deseeded and chopped
50g (2oz) fresh spinach leaves
3 tomatoes, chopped
3 cardamom pods
3 garlic cloves, chopped
2 teaspoons ground coriander (cilantro)
2 teaspoons curry powder
2 tablespoons fresh coriander (cilantro), chopped
1 onion, chopped
1 teaspoon ground ginger
1/2 teaspoon turmeric
400mls (14fl oz) coconut milk
1 tablespoon olive oil

SERVES 4

Method

Heat the oil in a large saucepan and add the onion. Cook for around 5 minutes. Add the tomatoes and herbs and spices and cook for 1 minute. Add the lentils, squash and coconut milk and cook for around 20 minutes. If you need to add more liquid just had some warm water or vegetable stock (broth). Add the spinach and stir well for around 2 minutes until it has wilted. Serve with brown rice and salad.

Meatballs & Roast Vegetables

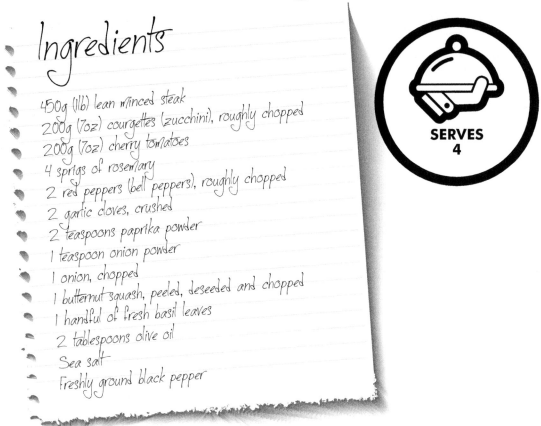

Ingredients

- 450g (1lb) lean minced steak
- 200g (7oz) courgettes (zucchini), roughly chopped
- 200g (7oz) cherry tomatoes
- 4 sprigs of rosemary
- 2 red peppers (bell peppers), roughly chopped
- 2 garlic cloves, crushed
- 2 teaspoons paprika powder
- 1 teaspoon onion powder
- 1 onion, chopped
- 1 butternut squash, peeled, deseeded and chopped
- 1 handful of fresh basil leaves
- 2 tablespoons olive oil
- Sea salt
- Freshly ground black pepper

SERVES 4

Method

Place the minced steak into a large bowl, add in the paprika and onion powder and mix well. Season with salt and pepper. Using clean hands, shape the meat into balls. Place the vegetables, garlic and basil into a large ovenproof dish or baking tray and drizzle olive oil over the top. Season with salt and pepper and lay the rosemary on top. Make spaces for the meatballs and add them. Cook in an oven, preheated to 200C/400F for around 25 minutes or until the meatballs are completely cooked. Serve and eat straight away.

Prawn Risotto

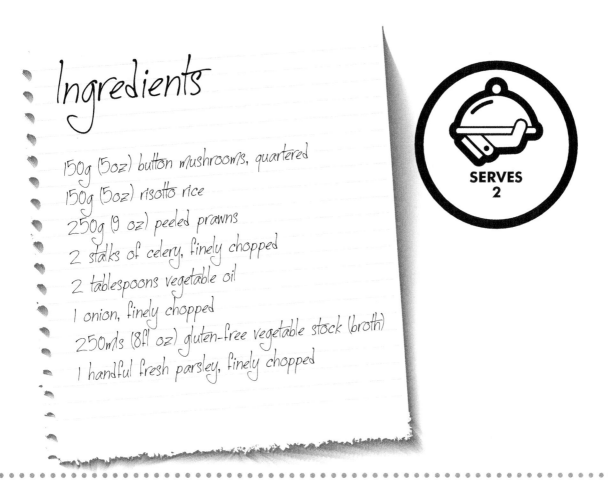

Ingredients

150g (5oz) button mushrooms, quartered

150g (5oz) risotto rice

250g (9 oz) peeled prawns

2 stalks of celery, finely chopped

2 tablespoons vegetable oil

1 onion, finely chopped

250mls (8fl oz) gluten-free vegetable stock (broth)

1 handful fresh parsley, finely chopped

SERVES 2

Method

Heat oil in a large frying, add the onions, celery and mushrooms and cook until they have softened. Add the risotto rice and prawns and stir. Pour in some of the vegetables stock (broth), gradually adding more as you stir. Once the rice has absorbed all of the liquid it should be creamy and soft. If you need to, you can add a little extra stock (or hot water). Stir in the parsley just before serving.

Coriander Chicken Stir-Fry

Ingredients

- 350g (12oz) brown rice
- 450 (1lb) chicken breasts, chopped
- 175g (6oz) mange tout (snow peas)
- 125g (4oz) broccoli, chopped
- 50g (2oz) fresh coriander leaves (cilantro)
- 4 garlic cloves, crushed
- 2.5cm (1 inch) chunk of fresh root ginger, peeled
- 2 teaspoons garam masala
- 1 green chilli, deseeded and finely chopped
- 1 onion, peeled and finely chopped
- ½ teaspoon chilli powder
- ½ teaspoon chilli flakes
- 2 tablespoons olive oil
- 2 teaspoons olive oil
- Juice of 1 lime
- A small handful of chopped fresh coriander (cilantro) for garnish

SERVES 4

Method

Place the coriander (cilantro), a teaspoon of olive oil, lime juice, ginger, chilli and garam masala into a blender and blitz until smooth. Begin cooking the rice according to the instructions. Heat 2 tablespoons of olive oil in a frying pan, add the onions, and garlic and cook for 5 minutes. Add in the chicken and brown it well. Add in the coriander (cilantro) mixture and continue cooking until the chicken is completely cooked through. Remove it and set aside, keeping it warm. Heat a teaspoon of olive oil in the frying pan and add in the chopped broccoli and mange tout. You can add a little warm water if you wish to keep it moist. Cook the vegetables for 4-5 minutes until they have softened. Return the chicken to the pan and stir. Add in the rice and mix well. Serve with a sprinkling of coriander.

Red Pepper Prawn Salad

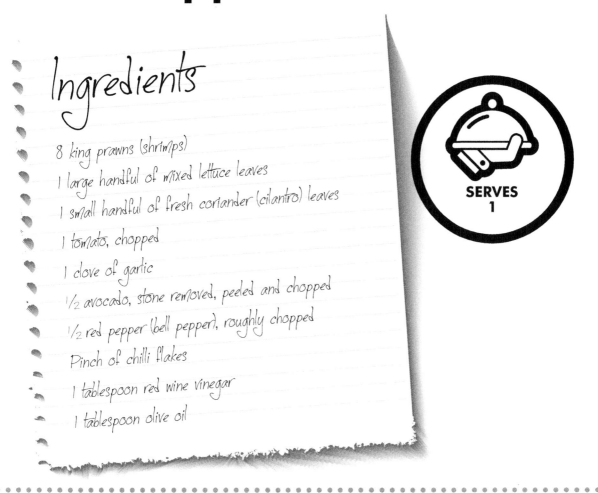

Ingredients

8 king prawns (shrimps)

1 large handful of mixed lettuce leaves

1 small handful of fresh coriander (cilantro) leaves

1 tomato, chopped

1 clove of garlic

1/2 avocado, stone removed, peeled and chopped

1/2 red pepper (bell pepper), roughly chopped

Pinch of chilli flakes

1 tablespoon red wine vinegar

1 tablespoon olive oil

SERVES 1

Method

Place the red pepper (bell pepper), garlic, vinegar, oil and chilli flakes into a blender and blitz until smooth. Transfer the mixture to a bowl and add the prawns (shrimps). Allow them to marinate for at least 30 minutes. Heat a frying pan on high, add the prawns (shrimps) and cook them for around 5 minutes, or until they are pink and cooked through. Scatter the lettuce leaves on a plate and add the coriander (cilantro) tomato and avocado. Spoon the prawns and the sauce over the top. Eat straight away.

Lemon Pork Loin & Roast Winter Vegetables

Ingredients

900g (2lb) boneless pork loin, fat removed where possible

800g (1 3/4lb) potatoes, peeled and quartered

3 parsnips, peeled roughly chopped

2 teaspoons dried mixed herbs

2 leeks, roughly chopped

1 medium butternut squash, peeled and roughly chopped

1 onion, cut into wedges

1 teaspoon mustard

1 tablespoon vegetable oil

1 tablespoon water

Salt and freshly ground black pepper

A handful of fresh thyme leaves, roughly chopped

Juice and zest of 1 lemon

SERVES 4-6

Method

Preheat your oven to 190°C/380F. In a bowl, combine the water, mustard, lemon juice and lemon zest. Place the pork into a roasting tin and spread the mustard marinade over pork, covering it completely. Take another roasting tin and scatter the leeks, potatoes, onion, parsnips and squash into the tin. Drizzle the vegetable oil over the top and sprinkle on the dried herbs. Place the pork into the oven and cook for around 1 hour, or until cooked through. You can test it with a skewer to see if it's done. Remove the pork and let it rest. Let the vegetables continue cooking for another 10 minutes. Scatter the fresh thyme through the vegetables. Season with salt and pepper. Slice the pork and serve it alongside the roast veggies. Enjoy.

Quinoa Salad

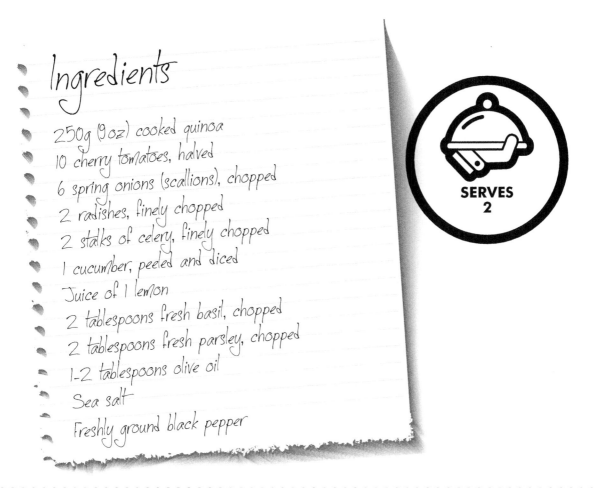

Ingredients

250g (9oz) cooked quinoa

10 cherry tomatoes, halved

6 spring onions (scallions), chopped

2 radishes, finely chopped

2 stalks of celery, finely chopped

1 cucumber, peeled and diced

Juice of 1 lemon

2 tablespoons fresh basil, chopped

2 tablespoons fresh parsley, chopped

1-2 tablespoons olive oil

Sea salt

Freshly ground black pepper

SERVES 2

Method

Place the quinoa, herbs and vegetables into a bowl and mix well. Drizzle the olive oil over the top and stir it through. Season with salt and pepper. Chill before serving.

Mediterranean Roast Chicken

Ingredients

6 sprigs of oregano, stalk removed

2 large handfuls of rocket (arugula) leaves

2 teaspoons dried mixed herbs or herbs de Provence

1 large whole chicken

1 sliced lemon

2 tablespoons olive oil

Juice of 2 lemons

Salt and pepper

Fresh oregano sprigs for garnish

SERVES 4

Method

Place the fresh oregano, dried herbs, lemon juice, olive oil, salt and pepper into a large bowl and mix well. Place the chicken into the marinade. Cover and chill in the fridge for at least 1 hour or overnight if you can. Place the chicken and marinade juices into a roasting tin and cook at 180C/360F for around 1½ hours, or until the juices of the chicken run clear when tested with a skewer. Carve the chicken and serve with slices of lemon and fresh rocket (arugula) leaves. Additionally you can serve the chicken with fresh steamed vegetables or roasted cauliflower.

Turkey & Sweet Potato Pie

Ingredients

600g (1lb 5oz) sweet potato, peeled and chopped

450g (1lb) minced (ground) turkey

400g (14oz) tin of chopped tomatoes

150g (5oz) frozen peas

3 celery stalks, finely chopped

1 onion, finely chopped

1 large carrot, peeled, finely chopped

2 tablespoons tomato purée (paste)

1 teaspoon dried mixed herbs

1 tablespoon olive oil

2 teaspoons Worcestershire sauce

Sea salt

Freshly ground black pepper

SERVES 4

Method

Heat the oil in a saucepan, add the carrot, onion and celery and cook gently for around 5 minutes until the vegetables have softened. Add the turkey mince and brown it for around 5 minutes. Stir in the tomato purée (paste), Worcestershire sauce, tomatoes, peas and herbs. Cook for around 20 minutes, stirring occasionally. In the meantime, boil the sweet potato in water for around 8-10 minutes or until it becomes tender. Drain off the excess water and mash the sweet potato until smooth. Season it with salt and pepper. Spoon the turkey mixture into an ovenproof dish then add the mashed sweet potato on top, smoothing it out to the sides. Transfer it to the oven and cook for 30 minutes at 180C/360F.

Chicken Strips

Ingredients

50g (2oz) ground almonds (almond flour/almond meal)

2 chicken breasts, cut into strips

1 egg, beaten

1/2 teaspoon ground cumin

1/2 teaspoon paprika

1/2 teaspoon sea salt

1/4 teaspoon freshly ground black pepper

1 tablespoon olive oil

SERVES 2

Method

Place the egg into a bowl and whisk it. In a separate bowl combine the ground almonds (almond flour/almond meal), paprika, cumin, salt and pepper. Dip each piece of chicken in the egg then dip it into the almond mixture. Lay the goujons onto a plate, taking care that they don't stick together. Heat the olive oil in a large frying pan and add the goujons. Cook for 6-8 minutes, turning once halfway through. Place them on kitchen paper to drain off excess oil. Can be eaten on their own or serve with guacamole, sour cream dip or garlic mayonnaise.

Tender Pork Curry

Ingredients

- 450g (1lb) pork steaks, cubed
- 400g (14oz) tinned chopped tomatoes
- 150g (5oz) broccoli, broken into florets
- 3 cloves garlic, minced
- 1 onion, chopped
- 1 green chilli, finely chopped
- 1 tablespoon curry powder
- 1 teaspoon ground ginger
- 1 teaspoon ground coriander (cilantro)
- 300mls (½ pint) gluten-free beef stock (broth)
- 1 tablespoon olive oil
- Sea salt
- Freshly ground black pepper

SERVES 4

Method

Heat the olive oil in a frying pan and add in the pork. Brown it for several minutes then transfer it to a slow cooker. Add in all the remaining ingredients and stir well. Cover the slow cooker and cook for around 6 hours or until the meat is tender. Serve with rice or roast vegetables.

Baked Salmon & Fennel

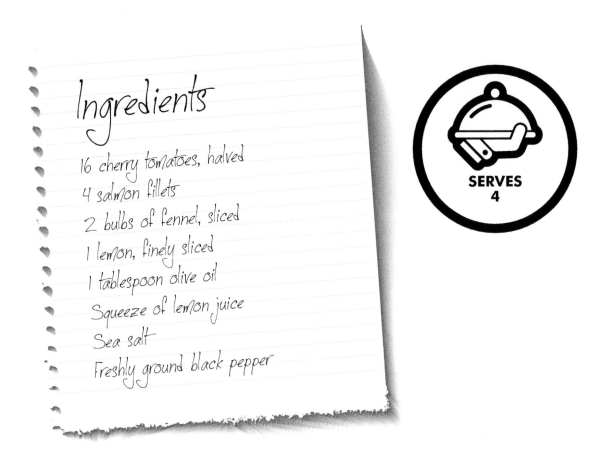

Ingredients

16 cherry tomatoes, halved

4 salmon fillets

2 bulbs of fennel, sliced

1 lemon, finely sliced

1 tablespoon olive oil

Squeeze of lemon juice

Sea salt

Freshly ground black pepper

SERVES 4

Method

Coat an ovenproof dish with the oil. Lay the slices of fennel and lemon on the dish and season with salt and pepper. Lay the salmon onto the bed of fennel. Squeeze a little lemon juice over it. Scatter the tomatoes on top. Cook for 13-15 minutes at 220C/430F or until the salmon is completely cooked through. Serve with a leafy salad and/or baby potatoes.

Lemon & Garlic King Prawns

Ingredients

SERVES 4

450g (1lb) raw king prawns (shrimps), shelled

20 cherry tomatoes

3 cloves of garlic, crushed

2 tablespoons fresh coriander (cilantro), chopped

1 yellow pepper (bell pepper), deseeded and roughly chopped

1 bag mixed lettuce leaves

2 tablespoons olive oil

Juice of 1 lemon

A lemon to garnish, quartered

Method

Place the garlic, lemon juice and olive oil into a bowl and mix well. Add in the prawns (shrimps), tomatoes and pepper and coat them in the mixture. Thread the ingredients alternately onto skewers. Place them under a hot grill (broiler) and cook until the vegetables have softened and the prawns are completely pink and cooked through. Scatter the mixed lettuce leaves onto plates and sprinkle with coriander (cilantro). Serve the prawns on top with a chunk of lemon. Enjoy straight away.

Thai Turkey Burger Wraps

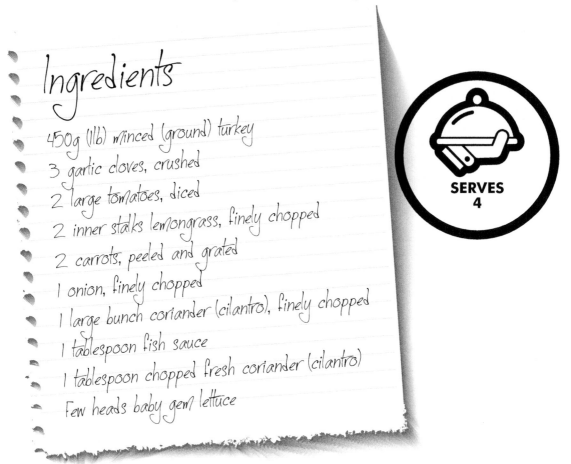

Ingredients

- 450g (1lb) minced (ground) turkey
- 3 garlic cloves, crushed
- 2 large tomatoes, diced
- 2 inner stalks lemongrass, finely chopped
- 2 carrots, peeled and grated
- 1 onion, finely chopped
- 1 large bunch coriander (cilantro), finely chopped
- 1 tablespoon fish sauce
- 1 tablespoon chopped fresh coriander (cilantro)
- Few heads baby gem lettuce

SERVES 4

Method

Place the turkey mince, garlic, coriander (cilantro), lemongrass, onion and fish sauce into a bowl and combine them well. Shape the mixture into balls then flatten them into round shapes. Place them on a lightly greased baking tray. Transfer them to the oven and bake at 200C/400F for 15–20 minutes. Meanwhile, you can make little salad boats to serve them in. In a bowl combine the chopped tomatoes with the grated carrots and a few sprigs of coriander (cilantro). Serve the turkey burgers into the lettuce leaves and add a spoonful of the tomato and carrot mixture into each one. Eat straight away. You could even add a little guacamole or mayonnaise to each one.

Harissa Chicken & Artichoke Salad

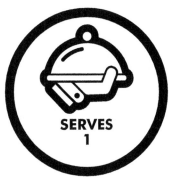

SERVES 1

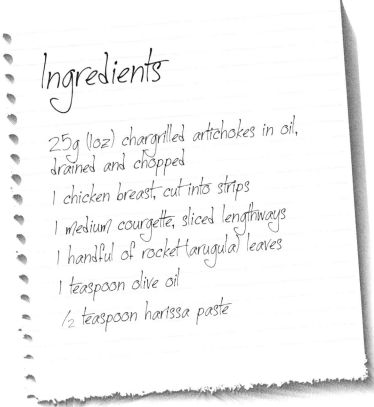

Ingredients

25g (1oz) chargrilled artichokes in oil, drained and chopped

1 chicken breast, cut into strips

1 medium courgette, sliced lengthways

1 handful of rocket (arugula) leaves

1 teaspoon olive oil

½ teaspoon harissa paste

Method

Place the harissa paste and olive oil in a bowl and coat the chicken in the mixture. Heat a griddle pan on a high heat and lay the courgette (zucchini) slices on it. Cook them until they have softened slightly then set them aside and keep warm. Place the chicken in the pan and cook it for around 6 minutes or until cooked completely, turning it over halfway through. Scatter the rocket (arugula) leaves onto a plate together with the artichoke pieces. Add the courgette and chicken to the salad. Serve and eat straight away.

Chilli Pork & Coriander Salsa

Ingredients

- 2 pork steaks
- 1 red chilli, de-seeded and chopped
- 2 tomatoes, peeled and de-seeded
- 2 tablespoons fresh coriander (cilantro), chopped
- 1/4 teaspoon chilli flakes
- 2 teaspoons red wine vinegar
- 1 tablespoon olive oil, for dressing
- 1 teaspoon olive oil, for frying
- Sea salt
- Freshly ground black pepper

SERVES 2

Method

Place the red chilli, tomatoes, coriander (cilantro), vinegar and oil into a bowl and mix well. Season with salt and pepper. Heat a teaspoon of olive oil in a frying pan. Sprinkle the chilli flakes onto the pork. Place the pork in the pan and cook for 5-6 minutes on each side or until it's completely cooked. Serve the salsa alongside. Enjoy.

Chicken & Vegetable Quinoa

Ingredients

175g (6oz) quinoa
4 medium chicken breasts, cut into strips
2 garlic cloves, finely chopped
2 tomatoes, diced
1 large courgette (zucchini), diced
1 onion, chopped
1 small handful of fresh basil leaves, chopped
450mls (15fl oz) gluten-free chicken stock (broth)
2 tablespoons olive oil
Juice of ½ lime

**SERVES
4**

Method

Place the quinoa and chicken stock (broth) into a large saucepan and boil it until the liquid is absorbed, usually around 12 minutes. The quinoa should be soft. Heat the oil in a frying pan, add the garlic and onion and cook until it softens. Add the chicken and cook it for around 8 minutes then set it aside. Add the courgette (zucchini) and tomato to the frying pan and cook for 5 minutes. Add the chicken back to the pan together with the lime and basil. Check that the chicken is completely cooked. Serve the quinoa onto plates then spoon the chicken and vegetables over the top. Enjoy straight away.

Speedy Mixed Bean Chilli

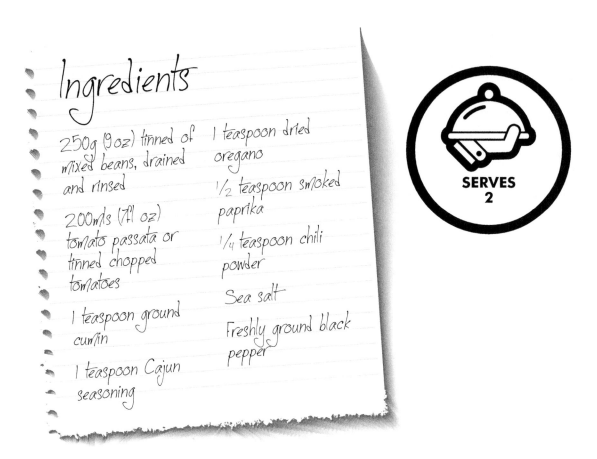

Ingredients

250g (9oz) tinned of mixed beans, drained and rinsed

200mls (7fl oz) tomato passata or tinned chopped tomatoes

1 teaspoon ground cumin

1 teaspoon Cajun seasoning

1 teaspoon dried oregano

1/2 teaspoon smoked paprika

1/4 teaspoon chili powder

Sea salt

Freshly ground black pepper

SERVES 2

Method

Place all of your ingredients into a saucepan, bring them to the boil and reduce the heat. Simmer for 10 minutes until the mixture is thoroughly warmed. Serve on its own along with a dollop of guacamole or with cauliflower rice, salsa and salad.

Creole Prawns

Ingredients

450g (1lb) peeled king prawns (shrimps)
250g (9oz) mange tout (snow peas)
2 x 400g (14oz) tinned chopped tomatoes
4 cloves garlic, chopped
1 tablespoon curry powder
1 teaspoon ground cumin
½ teaspoon paprika
200mls (7fl oz) gluten-free vegetable stock (broth)
3 tablespoons olive oil

**SERVES
4**

Method

Heat the oil in a frying pan, add the garlic, tomatoes, cumin, paprika, curry powder and stock (broth). Bring to the boil then reduce the heat and simmer for 10 minutes. Stir in the prawns (shrimps) mange tout (snow peas) and cook for around 10 minutes or until the prawns are cooked thoroughly and completely pink. Serve with brown rice.

Lemon & Spinach Chicken

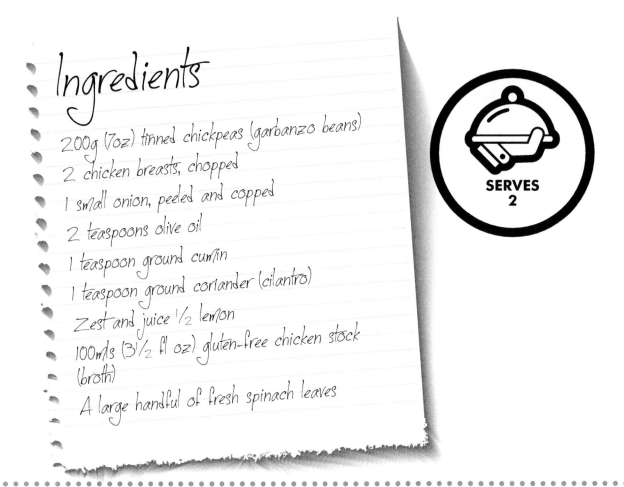

Ingredients

200g (7oz) tinned chickpeas (garbanzo beans)
2 chicken breasts, chopped
1 small onion, peeled and copped
2 teaspoons olive oil
1 teaspoon ground cumin
1 teaspoon ground coriander (cilantro)
Zest and juice ½ lemon
100mls (3½ fl oz) gluten-free chicken stock (broth)
A large handful of fresh spinach leaves

SERVES 2

Method

Heat the oil in a frying pan, add the onion and cook until it softens. Add in the chicken and cook for 4 minutes. Add in the cumin and coriander (cilantro) and stir well. Add in the chickpeas (garbanzo beans) and stock (broth). Cover the pan and cook for around 7 minutes. Add in the spinach and cook until it wilts. Stir in the lemon juice and zest. Serve and enjoy.

Sweet Potato Mash

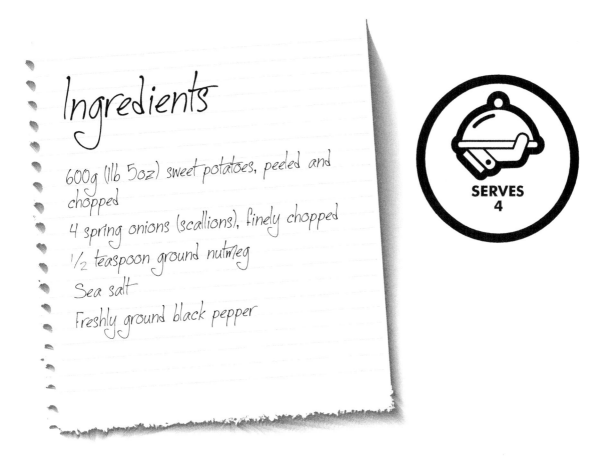

Ingredients

600g (1lb 5oz) sweet potatoes, peeled and chopped

4 spring onions (scallions), finely chopped

½ teaspoon ground nutmeg

Sea salt

Freshly ground black pepper

SERVES 4

Method

Place the sweet potatoes in a saucepan, bring them to the boil, reduce the heat and simmer for around 1 minutes or until the potatoes are soft. Drain the water off the sweet potatoes then mash them until there are no lumps left. Add the spring onions (scallions) and nutmeg and mix it well. Season and serve. These make a great alternative to the usual mashed potatoes.

Lamb & Red Pepper Skewers

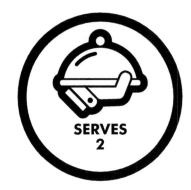

SERVES 2

Ingredients

250g (9oz) lean lamb steaks, cut into bite-sized chunks

1 tablespoon tomato purée (paste)

3 cloves of garlic, crushed

1 red pepper (bell pepper), cut into chunks

1 small red onion, cut into chunks

1/2 teaspoon onion powder

1 teaspoon smoked paprika

1 tablespoon olive oil

Method

Place the paprika, tomato purée (paste), onion powder, garlic and olive oil into a bowl and mix well. Add the lamb chunks and coat them well in the marinade. Cover them and let it marinate for at least an hour. Thread the meat, onion and pepper onto skewers, alternating the ingredients. Place the skewers under a pre-heated grill (broiler) and cook for 9-10 minutes, turning during cooking until the lamb is cooked through.

Lemon & Pine Nut Risotto

Ingredients

225g (8oz) risotto rice (arborio)

4 stalks of celery, finely chopped

3 tablespoons pine nuts

3 cloves of garlic, crushed

1 onion, finely chopped

1 tablespoon fresh parsley, chopped

1 tablespoon fresh coriander (cilantro), chopped

1/2 teaspoon sea salt

3 tablespoons olive oil

750mls (1½ pint) gluten-free vegetable stock (broth)

Zest and juice of 1 lemon

SERVES 4

Method

Heat the oil in a large saucepan, add the celery, onion and garlic and cook until the vegetables have softened. Add the rice, salt, lemon juice and zest. Pour the stock (broth) a little at a time during cooking, stirring occasionally, until the rice absorbs all of the stock. It's ready when the rice is soft and creamy, usually around 20 minutes. Stir in the pine nuts and herbs just before serving.

SNACKS & SWEET TREATS

Chocolate Mug Cake

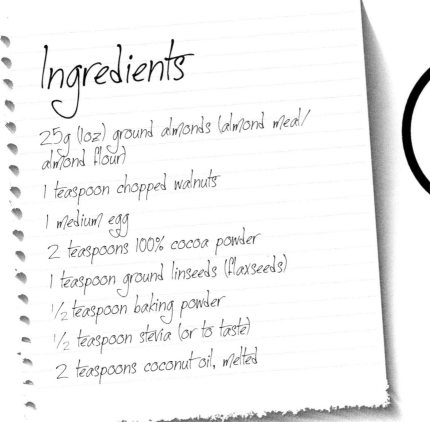

Ingredients

25g (1oz) ground almonds (almond meal/ almond flour)

1 teaspoon chopped walnuts

1 medium egg

2 teaspoons 100% cocoa powder

1 teaspoon ground linseeds (flaxseeds)

1/2 teaspoon baking powder

1/2 teaspoon stevia (or to taste)

2 teaspoons coconut oil, melted

SERVES 1

Method

Place all the ingredients, except the walnuts, into a large mug or a microwaveable bowl and mix well. Cook in the microwave for 30 seconds, remove and stir then return it to the microwave for another 30 seconds, remove and stir in the walnuts. Return it to the microwave for another 30 seconds. Can be served hot or cold, on its own or with a dollop of cream or coconut cream.

Choc-Chip & Banana Ice-Cream

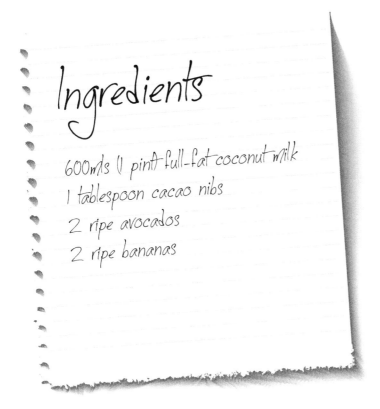

Ingredients

600mls (1 pint) full-fat coconut milk
1 tablespoon cacao nibs
2 ripe avocados
2 ripe bananas

Method

Place all the ingredients into a food processor or use a hand blender and blitz until smooth. Pour the mixture into an ice-cream maker and process according to the instructions for your model of machine. Serve straight away or freeze it. If you don't have an ice cream maker, place it in the freezer and occasionally whisk with a fork while it's freezing.

Homemade Almond Milk

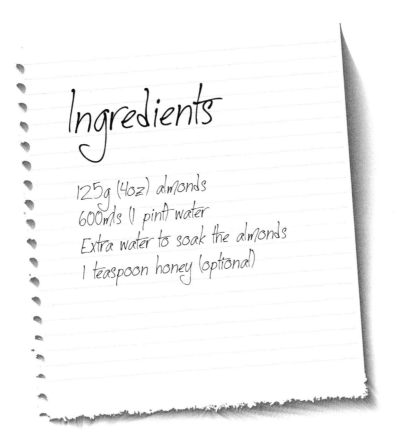

Ingredients

125g (4oz) almonds
600mls (1 pint) water
Extra water to soak the almonds
1 teaspoon honey (optional)

Method

Place the almonds into a bowl and cover them completely with water, covering them about 4cms (2 inches) deep. Cover the bowl and allow the almonds to soak overnight. Drain the water off the almonds and remove their skins. Rinse with cold water. Place the almonds into a food processor and add in 600mls (1 pint) of water. Blitz until the almonds are fine and the water is white and milky. Line a strainer or sieve with muslin cloth over a bowl and strain the almonds from the milk, squeezing the excess milk through the cloth. Stir in the honey, if using. Pour the milk into an airtight glass container and it will keep for2 to 3 days. Rather than waste the almonds, you can scatter them on a plate to dry them out and use them as you would ground almonds.

Poached Peaches

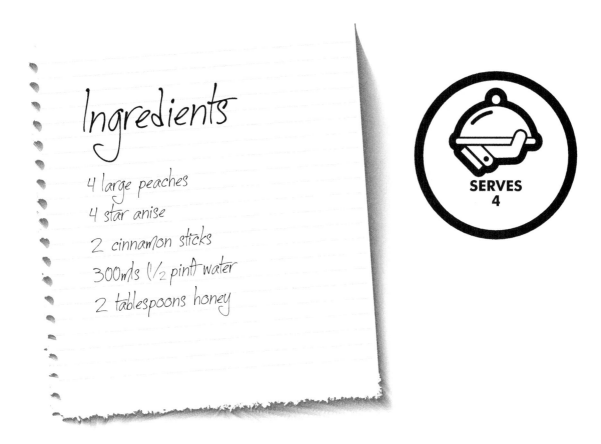

Ingredients

4 large peaches
4 star anise
2 cinnamon sticks
300mls (1/2 pint) water
2 tablespoons honey

SERVES 4

Method

Place the honey and water in a saucepan and bring to the boil. Add the peaches, star anise and cinnamon sticks. Reduce the heat and simmer gently for 10 minutes. Remove the peaches and set aside. Continue cooking the liquid for another 12-14 minutes until it begins to thicken. If necessary, return the peaches to the saucepan to warm them before serving.

Raspberry Chia Pudding

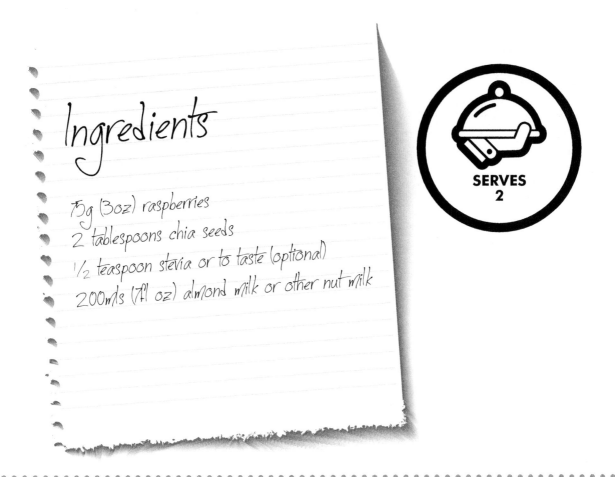

Ingredients

75g (3oz) raspberries
2 tablespoons chia seeds
½ teaspoon stevia or to taste (optional)
200mls (7fl oz) almond milk or other nut milk

SERVES 2

Method

Place the chia seeds, almond milk and stevia (if using) into a bowl and mix well. Cover them and place them in the fridge for 1-2 hours or overnight if you can. In the morning serve with a heap of raspberries over the top. Enjoy.

Banana Milkshake

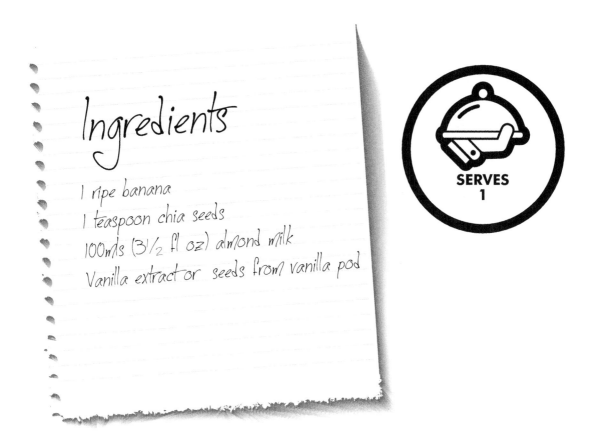

Ingredients

1 ripe banana
1 teaspoon chia seeds
100mls (3½ fl oz) almond milk
Vanilla extract or seeds from vanilla pod

**SERVES
1**

Method

Place all the ingredients into a food processor and mix until smooth and creamy.

Cinnamon Hot Chocolate

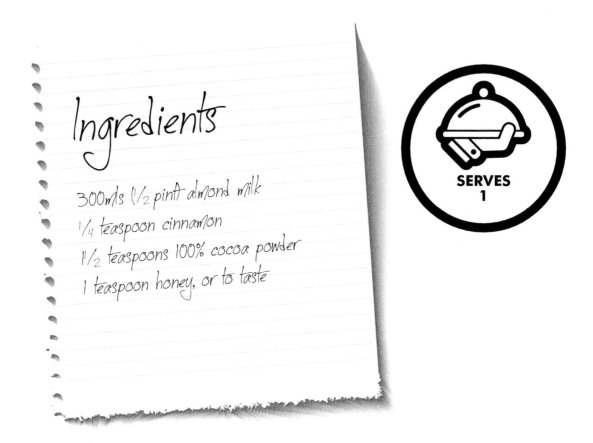

Ingredients

300mls (½ pint) almond milk

¼ teaspoon cinnamon

1½ teaspoons 100% cocoa powder

1 teaspoon honey, or to taste

SERVES
1

Method

Place all the ingredients into a saucepan and mix well. Place on a medium heat and warm the milk. Remove it from the heat and whisk it really well to make it frothy. Pour into your favourite mug.

Roast Pumpkin Seeds

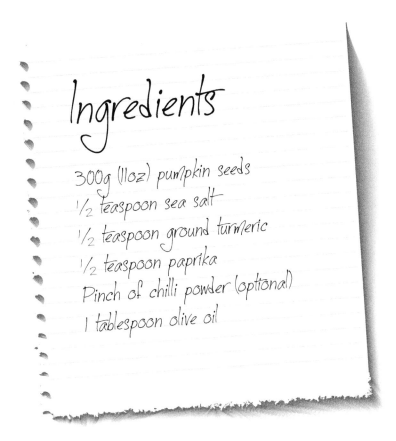

Ingredients

300g (11oz) pumpkin seeds
1/2 teaspoon sea salt
1/2 teaspoon ground turmeric
1/2 teaspoon paprika
Pinch of chilli powder (optional)
1 tablespoon olive oil

Method

Place the pumpkin seeds into a bowl and stir in the olive oil, salt, paprika, chilli powder (if using) and turmeric. Scatter the pumpkin seeds onto a baking tray. Place them into an oven, preheated to 140C/ 280F for around 15 minutes. Remove them from the oven and let them cool. Store them in an airtight container until ready to use.

Cinnamon Spiced Almonds

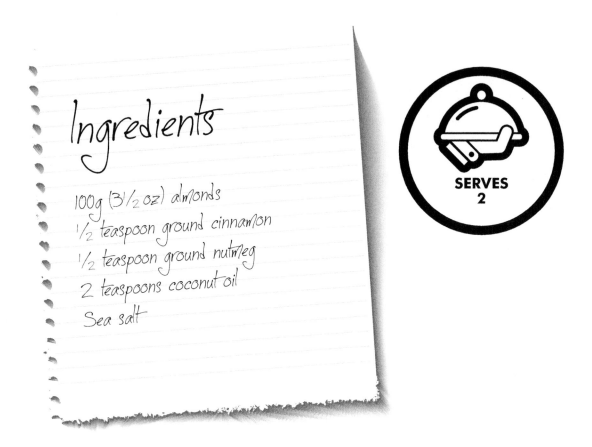

Ingredients

100g (3½ oz) almonds
½ teaspoon ground cinnamon
½ teaspoon ground nutmeg
2 teaspoons coconut oil
Sea salt

SERVES 2

Method

Heat the coconut oil in a large frying pan. Add the almonds, cinnamon, nutmeg and salt. Stir constantly for around 7-8 minutes. Allow them to cool before eating. You can also increase the batch size and store some in an airtight container.

You may also be interested in other titles by
Erin Rose Publishing
which are available in both paperback and ebook.

Quick Start Guides

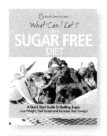
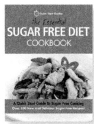
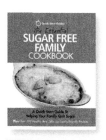
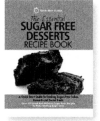
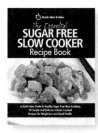
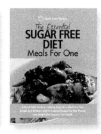

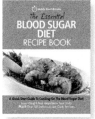
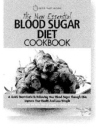
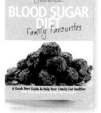
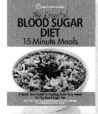
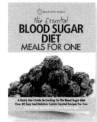
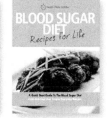

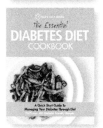
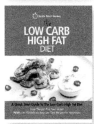
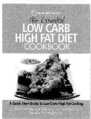
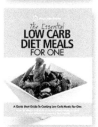
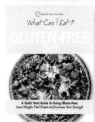
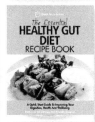

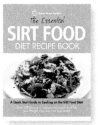
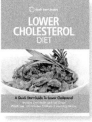
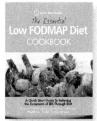
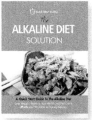

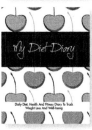
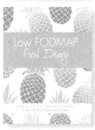
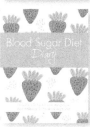
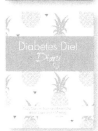
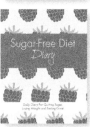

Books by Sophie Ryan
Erin Rose Publishing

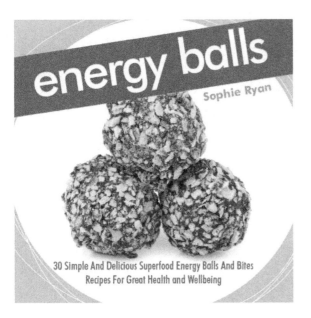

30 Simple And Delicious Superfood Energy Balls And Bites
Recipes For Great Health and Wellbeing

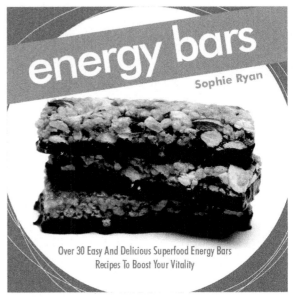

Over 30 Easy And Delicious Superfood Energy Bars
Recipes To Boost Your Vitality

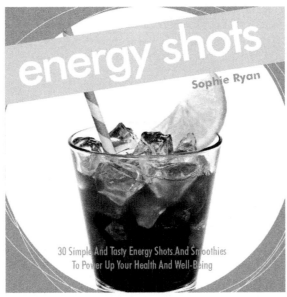

30 Simple And Tasty Energy Shots And Smoothies
To Power Up Your Health And Well-Being

Printed in Great Britain
by Amazon